HAND PAIN
and Impairment

HAND PAIN
and Impairment
EDITION 4

RENE CAILLIET, M.D.

Professor and Chairman Emeritus
Department of Physical Medicine and Rehabilitation
School of Medicine
University of Southern California
Los Angeles, California

Illustrations by R. Cailliet, M.D.

 F.A. DAVIS COMPANY · Philadelphia

F. A. Davis Company
1915 Arch Street
Philadelphia, PA 19103

Printed in the United States of America

Last digit indicates print number: 10 9 8 7 6 5 4 3 2 1

Note: As new scientific information becomes available through basic and clinical research, recommended treatments and drug therapies undergo changes. The author and publisher have done everything possible to make this book accurate, up-to-date, and in accord with accepted standards at the time of publication. The author, editors, and publisher are not responsible for errors or omissions or for consequences from application of the book, and make no warranty, expressed or implied, in regard to the contents of the book. Any practice described in this book should be applied by the reader in accordance with professional standards of care used in regard to the unique circumstances that may apply in each situation. The reader is advised always to check product information (package inserts) for changes and new information regarding dose and contraindications before administering any drug. Caution is especially urged when using new or infrequently ordered drugs.

Library of Congress Cataloging-in-Publication Data

Cailliet, Rene.
    Hand pain and impairment / Rene Cailliet ; illustrations by R.
Cailliet. — Ed. 4.
        p.   cm.
    Includes bibliographical references and index.
    ISBN 0-8036-1619-8
    1. Hand—Diseases.   2. Pain.   I. Title.
    [DNLM: 1. Hand.   2. Hand Injuries—therapy.   3. Pain—therapy.
WE 830 C134h   1994]
RC951.C24   1994
617.5'75—dc20
DNLM/DLC
for Library of Congress   93-46466
                                                                      CIP

Preface

Since the publication of the third edition in 1983, there have been valuable additions to the understanding of the functional anatomy and pathophysiology of hand problems, prompting this new edition. Nowhere else in the human body is a thorough understanding of functional anatomy so important as in the hand; this forms the basis for an understanding of normal function and recognition of abnormal function. This new edition enhances this understanding by describing and illustrating proper techniques of clinical examination, based on both functional and gross anatomy.

In Chapter 1, Functional Anatomy, the previous edition had 50 illustrations; in this edition, there are 87. The techniques of examination are highlighted. Pathophysiology, which has been a field of constant, ongoing research, is highlighted throughout this edition. The fourth edition is totally current in all aspects, including surgical procedures, although these are not described in technical detail.

As in all the books on musculoskeletal disease in this series, the purpose of this volume is to educate all primary physicians to become medical orthopedists, to ensure that all patients with musculoskeletal injuries or illnesses have their problems recognized. All pertinent therapy thereupon evolves so that meaningful treatment protocols are based on an understanding of neuromusculoskeletal physiological concepts.

The sections on spasticity, burns, infections, and bracing have been enlarged and made current. The reference list, minimal in previous editions, has been expanded.

Therapists — physical, occupational, and vocational — and nurse practitioners will benefit from understanding these concepts as well as having therapeutic modalities fully discussed. A meaningful prescription for therapy should result in a benefit to all, especially the patient.

The hand is a precise, dexterous mechanism that defies casual understanding. Its functional loss is a major calamity in all aspects of life. Early thorough evaluation ensures a more complete recovery of function.

Rene Cailliet, MD

Contents

Illustrations

CHAPTER 1

Functional Anatomy

The hand is a complex functional portion of human anatomy that differentiates us from other species. It is an organ of fine sensation, discrimination, and exquisite dexterity. In conjunction with speech, hand function dominates mankind's cerebral cortical function.

A thorough knowledge of functional anatomy is vital to an understanding of the working of the hand, more so than for any other portion of the human anatomy. Nowhere in man is the term "neuromusculoskeletal" more applicable to function than in the hand.

The hand is placed in its functional position by coordinated action of the shoulder, upper arm, elbow, and forearm. The decision to use a precise hand function determines the numerous functions and positions of the entire upper extremity.

INSPECTION

Any evaluation of a hand must consider comparison with the contralateral and allegedly normal hand.

Clinical evaluation begins by general inspection and observation of three main actions: forming a fist, opening the entire hand, and spreading the fingers (Fig. 1–1). A further test of the hand is to have the patient "pinch" the tip of the thumb to the tip of the index finger and then to pinch the palmar surfaces of these two finger together (Fig. 1–2). These gross movements make it apparent that all joints move and that all required nerve controls are present.

The hand should be observed as the patient enters the examining room and awaits examination. The resting hand (Fig. 1–3) finds the

1

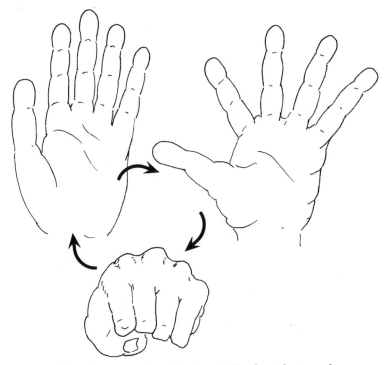

Figure 1–1. General examination of the hand. The fist at bottom shows a normal metacarpal arch and all fingers flexed at all joints with adequate rotation of the fingers. The open hand indicates that all joints of the fingers extend, implying adequate function of the nerve supply, full capsular flexibility, adequate flexibility of the skin, and functional extensor tendons. The thenar and hypothenar eminences also reveal the fullness of these muscles. The palmar skin shows no fibrous thickening. The open hand with fingers spread demonstrates adequate intrinsic muscles, competent articular joints of all fingers, normal motor nerve supply of the intrinsic muscles, and flexible web spaces between the fingers. Viewing the dorsum of the hand in these three actions permits viewing the nails and dorsal skin condition.

wrist slightly extended, the proximal phalanx flexed 15°, the middle phalanx flexed 60°, and the distal phalanx 15° (Fig. 1–4).

Cutaneous Covering

Tactile sensation and discrimination are important to ensure precise, dexterous motor activity of the hand. The skin plays a major role in this function.

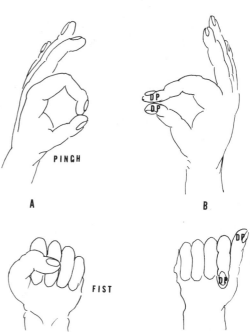

Figure 1-2. Anterior interosseous syndrome. The motor deficit of the anterior interosseous nerve syndrome causes inability to flex the distal phalanges (DP) of the index finger and thumb. The normal pinch (*upper A*) with tip to tip opposition is not possible (*upper B*) with the distal phalanges extended. In making a fist (*lower A*) the normally flexed fingers cannot flex at the index and thumb distal phalanges (*lower B*).

PINCH

A

B

FIST

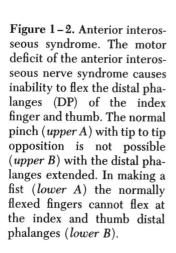

FINGERS FLEXED

WRIST DORSIFLEXED

INDEX–MIDDLE OPPOSED TO THUMB

THUMB ABDUCTED

Figure 1-3. The resting hand attitude. The resting hand and wrist "attitude" is with the wrist slightly extended and the proximal, middle, and distal phalanges slightly flexed. The thumb is slightly abducted and its phalanges are flexed.

Figure 1-4. Position of immobilization of finger joints in treatment of fractures. Immobilization of the joints of the fingers in treatment of fractures is best done with 15° of flexion at the metacarpophalangeal joint, 60° at the proximal interphalangeal joint, and 15° at the distal joint.

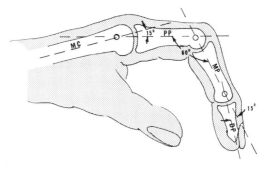

The volar and dorsal skin covering of the hand play a unique role in hand function. The dorsal skin is fine, supple, and mobile allowing full flexion of the digits. The dorsal skin contains hair follicles that play a tactile role and reinforce the protection of the underlying tissues.

The volar (palmar) skin, unlike the dorsal skin, is thick, hairless, inelastic, contains sweat glands, and is richly supplied with sensory nerve receptors. To facilitate uninhibited flexion, the skin contains numerous lines and creases. The skin is attached to the underlying palmar fascia.

Fascia

Fascia is an elastic collagen connective tissue that forms divisions containing muscles, nerves, blood vessels, lymphatics, and bones. Fascia is generally divided into superficial and deep layers, with the former being deep to the skin. In the hand (Fig. 1–5) it divides into three zones: central, lateral, and medial. The apex of the central zone is a continuation of the transverse carpal ligament. Distally, the central superficial palmar fascia divides into slips extending into each finger. The central fascia covers the flexor digitorum superficialis, flexor digitorum profundus, the terminal portion of the median nerve, and the superficial branch of the ulnar nerve.

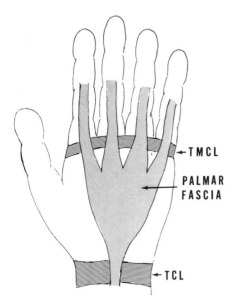

←TMCL

PALMAR FASCIA

←TCL

Figure 1–5. Palmar aponeurosis (fascia). The palmar fascia is schematically shown. TMCL = transverse metacarpal ligament; TCL transverse carpal ligament.

The medial aponeurosis and the lateral aponeurosis cover the thenar and the hypothenar eminences respectively. The deep palmar aponeurosis covers the floor of the palm between the two eminences and covers the interossei. Figure 4–20, page 180, depicts the normal anatomy of the palmar fascia.

Normally the palmar and dorsal fascia function to protect, cushion, and restrain the palm, and to conform to and maintain its convexity.[1]

The Palmar Surface

The palmar aspect of the hand and its wrinkles are examined to evaluate the status of the skin and underlying fascia (Fig. 1–6). The palmar creases exist at the sites of flexion of the joints of the hand. The major palmar creases are:

1. The distal palmar crease overlying the metacarpophalangeal joints.
2. The proximal palmar crease overlying the base of the fingers.
3. The proximal interphalangeal crease overlying the proximal interphalangeal joints.
4. The thenar crease outlining the thenar muscles and the proximal phalangealcarpal joint of the thumb.
5. The wrist crease where the proximal row of carpal bones articulates with the distal radius.
6. Interphalangeal creases at the distal phalanges and the middle interphalangeal joints.

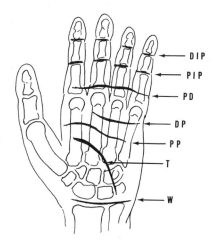

Figure 1–6. The palmar creases and their bony landmarks. DIP = distal interphalangeal crease; PIP = proximal interphalangeal crease; PD = palmar digital crease; DP = distal palmar crease; PP = proximal palmar crease; T = thenar crease; W = wrist crease.

The muscles within the palm lend themselves to gross examination by comparing the thenar and hypothenar eminences. The former is comprised of the muscles of the thumb and the latter of the muscles of the little finger.

In Figure 1–7 are shown the underlying bones forming the arches over which reside the thenar and hypothenar muscles, and forming the curves of the resting hand. The valley between the two eminences is the site of flexor tendons, neurovascular bundles upon a base formed by the carpal bones.

The Dorsal Surface

On viewing the fist (Fig. 1–1) one sees the hills and dales of the knuckles: the metacarpal heads residing over the transverse metacarpal arch (see Fig. 1–7), and the space between the heads.

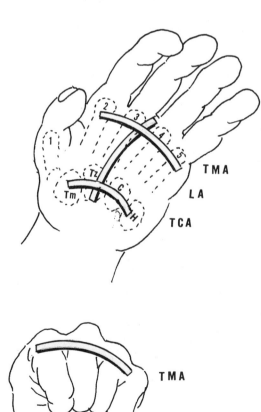

Figure 1–7. Arches of the hand: transverse and longitudinal. The upper drawing depicts the two transverse arches: the transverse metacarpal arch (TMA) and the transverse carpal arch (TCA), as well as the longitudinal arch (LA). The bottom drawing depicts the fist, showing the transverse metacarpal arch. The bones forming the arches are the metacarpals, numbered 1 through 5, and the carpal bones: the hamate (H), capitate (C), trapezium (Tm), and trapezoid (Tz).

The skin of the dorsum contains hair follicles and is coarser than the palmar skin. Observe the nails for shape: (spoon [concave] or clubbed [convex]) and color can reveal the status of the circulatory system locally or generally.

The skin of the palmar region is firmly attached to the underlying fascia, permitting firm gripping of objects, whereas the dorsal skin is freer. The dorsal skin normally can be grasped between the fingers of the examiner and elevated and moved. As there are significant underlying venous and lymphatic fluid channels on the dorsum, edema of the hand is observed first on the dorsum of the fingers. The dorsal skin must also be flexible to allow full flexion of each entire finger.

BONY PALPATION

There are 29 bones forming the hand and wrist (Fig. 1–8). The history of a patient may indicate the cause and the site of pain, as well as the nature of the functional loss, but a careful, precise examination of each of the component bones involved is needed to ascertain the diagnosis.

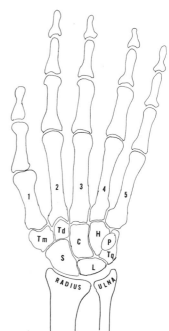

Figure 1–8. Bones of the hand. The composite of the bones of the left hand viewed from the palmar surface. The proximal row contains the (navicular) scaphoid (S), lunate (L), and triquetrum (Tq). The distal row contains the trapezium (greater multangular; Tm), trapezoid (lesser multangular; Td), capitate, and hamate. The pisiform (P) is considered to be in the proximal row.

Wrist

The wrist joint, termed the carpus, is the articulation between the forearm and the carpal bones. There are eight carpal bones situated in two rows. The proximal row from the radial (thumb) side contains the navicular (scaphoid), the lunate, the triquetrum, and (anterior to the triquetrum) the pisiform bones. The distal row from the radial side contains the trapezium (greater multangular), the trapezoid (lesser multangular), the capitate, and the hamate bones (Fig. 1–9).

The bones of the forearm, the radius and the ulna, form the proximal row of the wrist and end with styloid processes. With the palm facing up, the radial styloid is lateral. It usually reaches further distally than does the ulnar styloid, although in 60 percent of the population the projections of the processes are equal. The dorsal surface is longer (distally) than is the volar (Fig. 1–10).

The distal end of the radius is concave and articulates with the curvature of the proximal carpal row in an incongruous manner, that is, the curvatures are not symmetrical. The radio-ulnar surface is less concave than the curve of the proximal carpal row. This is also true from a lateral view, in which the curvatures are also incongruous. The obliquity of the radial and ulnar styloids causes the hand to rest in a slightly ulnar and palmar posture (Fig. 1–11).

There are two facets on the distal surface of the radius (Fig. 1–12). The scaphoid bone glides upon the triangular radial facet, and the lunate glides upon the cuboid facet. Wrist movements are oblique gliding motions, with the carpal row gliding upon the cartilage of the radial surface.

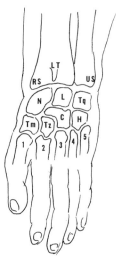

Figure 1–9. Bones forming the wrist (dorsal view). The radial bone with the radial styloid (RS) and the ulnar styloid (US) form the proximal wall of the wrist. Lister's tubercle (LT) is found on the dorsum of the radius. The radial styloid is slightly more distal than is the ulnar styloid. The proximal row of carpal bones are the navicular (N), lunate (L) and triquetrum (Tq), which articulate with the distal row of the trapezium (Tm), the trapezoid (Tz), the capitate (C), and the hamate (H). The five metacarpal heads (1–5) articulate with the distal carpal row.

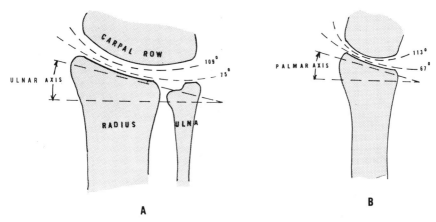

A   **B**

Figure 1 – 10. Relationship of the carpal row to the radioulnar surface. (*A*) The radial margin of the radius protrudes further than does the ulnar side. The articular surface is thus on an oblique plane. (*B*) The dorsal edge protrudes further than the palmar (volar) margin. The joint surfaces are incongruous; the carpal row is more convex than the opposing surface of the radius.

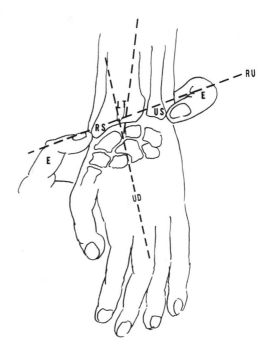

Figure 1 – 11. Obliquity of the radial ulnar styloids. The radial styloid (RS) protrudes further distally than does the ulnar styloid (US), forming an oblique radial-ulnar line (RU). Both are palpable by the examiner (E), as is the Lister tubercle (LT). The obliquity causes the resting hand to face in an ulnar deviation (UD) and in a flexed position.

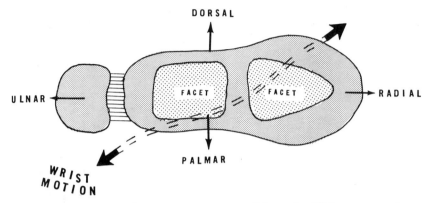

Figure 1–12. Functional movement patterns of the wrist. Wrist movements are not in one plane. All the muscles across the wrist act *obliquely*. Therefore, wrist movement is radiodorsal to ulnar-palmar. This plane of wrist movement is due to antagonistic muscle group pairing—extensor carpi radialis versus flexor carpi ulnaris and the long flexors of the fingers.

As the hand abducts in a radial direction, the proximal carpal row glides in an ulnar direction (Fig. 1–13); the opposite occurs in abduction towards the ulnar side.

Ligaments controlling the wrist motions include the longitudinal, radial, and ulnar ligaments, plus the transverse and oblique ligaments (Fig. 1–14). As with all ligamentous structures, they become taut to limit motion, and slack, in the opposite direction, to permit motion.

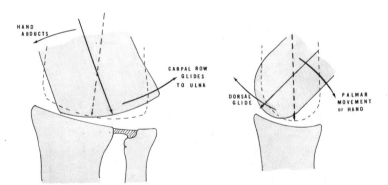

Figure 1–13. Gliding motion of the carporadial articulation. The motion between the radial surface and the proximal carpal row is that of gliding. The carpal bones glide in the direction opposite from the hand's movements. This gliding movement is permitted by capsular and ligamentous laxity.

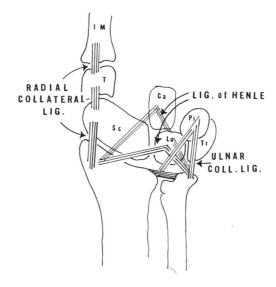

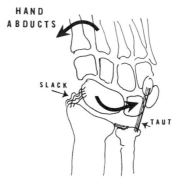

Figure 1–14. Ligaments of the wrist. The ulnar and radial collateral and the dorsal and palmar oblique ligaments support the wrist. Radial deviation of the hand tightens the ulnar collateral ligaments; ulnar deviation tightens the radial ligaments.

The ulnar collateral ligament arises from the ulnar styloid process and the triangular ligament attaching to the pisiform bone. It becomes taut when the hand deviates radially. The radial collateral ligament arises from the radial styloid process, attaches to the scaphoid, and passes on to the trapezium and first metacarpal. It becomes taut when the hand deviates in an ulnar direction. The examiner can evaluate the integrity of these ligaments by moving the hand in both directions.

The transverse-oblique wrist ligaments on the palmar surface maintain the carpal arch (see Fig. 1–7). The palmar ulnar and palmar radiocarpal ligaments converge at the midline to attach to the lunate and capitate bones and form the arcuate ligament of Henle. The dorsal ligaments are less symmetrical and more lax. Supination of the hand tightens the palmar ligaments, and pronation tightens the dorsal ligaments.

The active and passive range of motion of the wrist is determined in a clinical examination, and the abnormal wrist is compared to the normal (Fig. 1–15). Passive range of motion occurs in flexion and extension, but there are, in addition, joint motions, not under voluntary control and present in all normal joints, called "joint play."[2,3] (See Fig. 1–16.) The motions involved in joint play are traction (separation), translation in a dorsal and palmar direction, and rotation about the

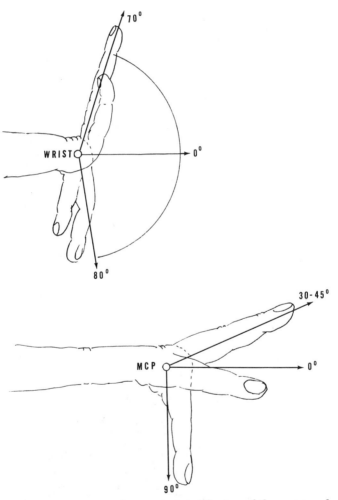

Figure 1–15. Measurement of extension and flexion of the wrist and metacarpophalangeal joints. The normal ranges of wrist extension (70°) and flexion (80°) are derived from neutral (0°). The ranges of metacarpophalangeal joint motion are also stated as 30° to 45° extension and 90° flexion.

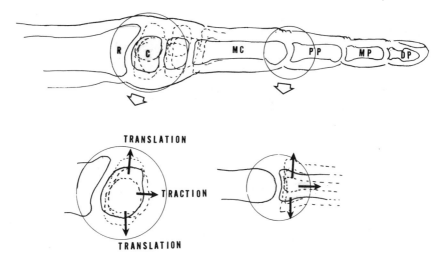

Figure 1–16. Joint play. Every joint in the body has joint play, which indicates possible passive movement other than flexion and extension. In this drawing the play is shown between the carpal bones (C) and the radius (R), and between the metacarpal (MC) and the proximal phalanx (PP). The joint play implies capsular laxity that permits traction of the distal from the proximal bone and translation dorsally and volarly. The dotted outlines indicate the newly gained position of the bone after applications of the forces.

longitudinal axis. They are elicited by the examiner upon manipulation of the patient's specific joint. Adequate joint play is necessary, as all joints not only flex and extend but, being incongruous, must glide.[4]

Carpal Bones

The eight carpal bones are arranged in two rows, each bone having a cuboid shape with six surfaces. The four surfaces that articulate with other carpal bones are covered with cartilage. The two other surfaces, the dorsal and volar, are roughened for ligamentous attachments.

The proximal carpal row contains the scaphoid, lunate, and triquetrum (Fig. 1–17). A fourth bone, the pisiform bone, is on the palmar surface of the triquetrum and thus is considered to be a sesamoid bone and not one of the proximal row. The proximal carpal row articulates with the radius, forming the wrist joint.

The distal carpal row contains the os trapezium (greater multangular), os trapezoid (lesser multangular), the capitate, and the hamate bones. The distal border of the proximal carpal row is concave and

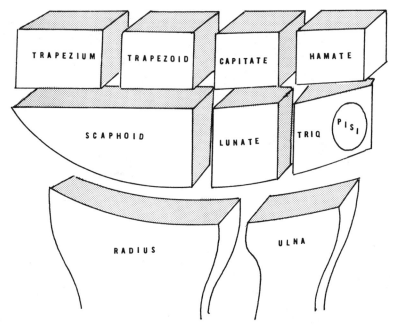

Figure 1–17. Carpal bones (schematic). The left hand is viewed from the palmar surface.

articulates with the convex proximal border of the distal row. The trapezium and trapezoid articulate with the scaphoid, capitate, and lunate bones, and the hamate with the triquetrum. No carpal bone articulates with the ulna.

In palmar flexion and dorsal extension of the hand, the distal carpal row glides upon the proximal row, with a greater degree of flexion occurring at the radiocarpal joints (see Fig. 1–13). In extension (dorsal flexion), most movement occurs in the midcarpal joints, with less occurring at the radiocarpal joint.

Radial deviation occurs mostly in the midcarpal joints, with ulnar deviation occurring mostly at the radiocarpal joint. In radial abduction of the hand, the proximal row moves in an ulnar direction. The distal row moves in an ulnar direction upon the proximal row (Fig. 1–18).

In ulnar hand deviation, the capitate moves towards the radial side and disengages from the proximal row. The scaphoid bone moves the greatest distance—approximately 1 cm. The ligaments of the wrist (see Fig. 1–14) support the structure and limit the movement.

The carpal bones are "close packed" for stability and are reinforced by the intercarpal ligaments (Fig. 1–19).

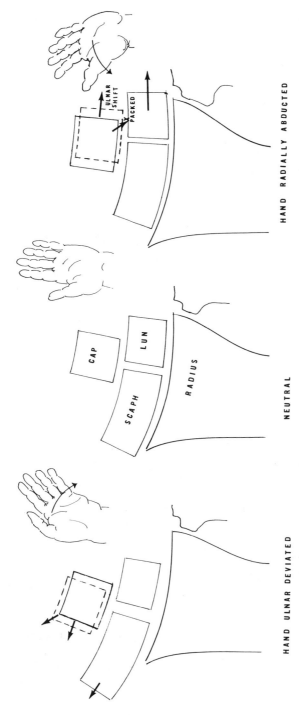

Figure 1–18. Carpal movement. When the hand moves radially, the carpal rows move in the opposite (ulnar) direction. The capitate glides ulnarly and *toward* the proximal row to pack tight. In ulnar movement of the hand, the opposite occurs.

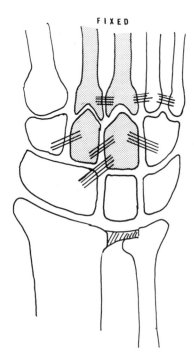

FIXED

Figure 1–19. Intercarpal ligaments. The dorsal ligaments are related. The palmar ligaments shown here are transverse in their direction radiating principally from the capitate. There are few ligaments between the proximal and distal carpal rows.

In addition to the intercarpal ligaments, the palmar arch is maintained by the transverse carpal ligament (Fig. 1–20), which is comprised of two bands: a proximal and a distal.

The proximal band is attached to the tubercle of the navicular bone and extends to the pisiform bone (Fig. 1–21), which can be considered a sesamoid bone within the tendon. As the pisiform is a mobile bone, this band may be relaxed, but becomes taut when the flexor carpi ulnaris muscle is contracted, as when the hand is held in an ulnar flexed position. The distal band of the transverse carpal ligament is always taut, being attached to two fixed points: the tubercle of the trapezium and the hook of the hamate.

The concavity of the arched carpal bones is bridged by the transverse ligaments, forming the "carpal tunnel". (Fig. 1–22) This tunnel is deep enough to permit the insertion of a fingertip, if all its contents were removed.

The tunnel contains the tendons of the flexor digitorum profundus, which lie upon both the carpal bones and their intercarpal ligaments, and, more superficially, the flexor digitorum superficialis tendons. Also within the tunnel are found the flexor carpi radialis and the flexor pollicis longus tendons, as well as the median nerve.

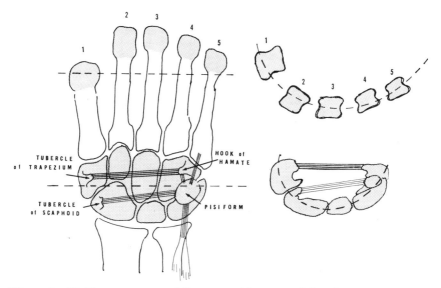

Figure 1–20. Transverse carpal ligament. Also termed the *flexor retinaculum*, this ligament bridges the arch of the carpal rows. It is formed by two bands — the proximal, extending from the tubercle of scaphoid to the pisiform, and the distal band, from the tubercle of the trapezium to the hook of the hamate.

Clinical Evaluation of the Carpal Bones

The superficial landmarks of the structures involved at the palmar aspect of the wrist are shown in Figure 1–23. The distal skin crease of the wrist corresponds to the proximal border of the transverse carpal ligament. The flexor carpi radialis leads to the tubercle of the scaphoid and can be palpated when the clenched fist is flexed and radially abducted against resistance (Fig. 1–24).

The radial artery can be palpated on the radial side between the tendon of the flexor carpi radialis and the abductor pollicis longus. The ulnar artery is palpable just to the radial side of the flexor carpi ulnaris tendon. The radial artery is readily palpable, whereas the ulnar artery lies too deep under a thick fascia to be easily palpable.

Clinical Evaluation by Bony Palpation

Clinical evaluation of the wrists and therefore of the carpal bones begins by gross examination of the wrists in dorsiflexion and palmar flexion (Fig. 1–25). Since trauma may involve the carpal bones, clinical examination requires that each bone precisely examined. Carpal bones may dislocate. (Fig. 1–26) as determined by their configuration.

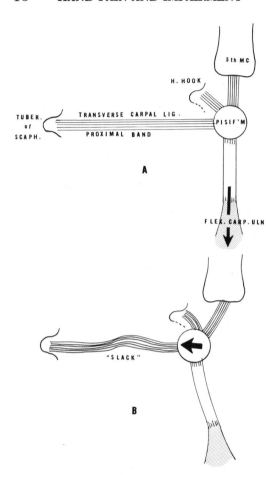

Figure 1–21. Proximal band of transverse carpal ligament. This structure is taut or slack depending upon the tension on the pisiform by the flexor carpi ulnaris. The pisiform is a sesamoid bone within the tendon of the flexor carpi ulnaris, which attaches to the base of the fifth metacarpal and the hook of the hamate. (A) The contracted muscle tenses the transverse ligament. (B) Both are slack.

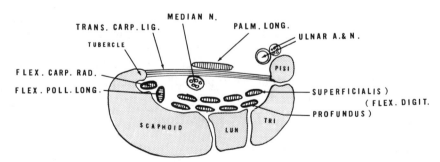

Figure 1–22. Carpal tunnel contents. The tunnel formed by the carpal bones and the spanning transverse carpal ligament contains the tendons of the long finger flexors (deep and superficial), tendons of the flexor pollicis longus and flexor carpi radialis, and the median nerve.

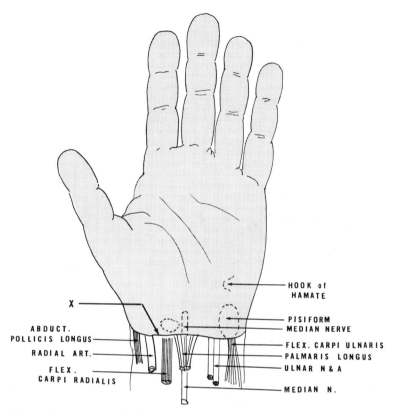

HOOK of HAMATE

X

PISIFORM

ABDUCT. POLLICIS LONGUS

MEDIAN NERVE

RADIAL ART.

FLEX. CARPI ULNARIS

PALMARIS LONGUS

FLEX. CARPI RADIALIS

ULNAR N & A

MEDIAN N.

Figure 1–23. Superficial landmarks at the palmar surface of the wrist.

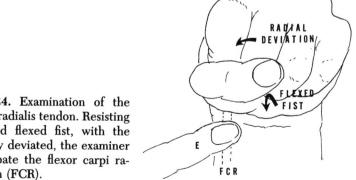

RADIAL DEVIATION

FLEXED FIST

E

FCR

Figure 1–24. Examination of the flexor carpi radialis tendon. Resisting the clenched flexed fist, with the hand radially deviated, the examiner (E) can palpate the flexor carpi radialis tendon (FCR).

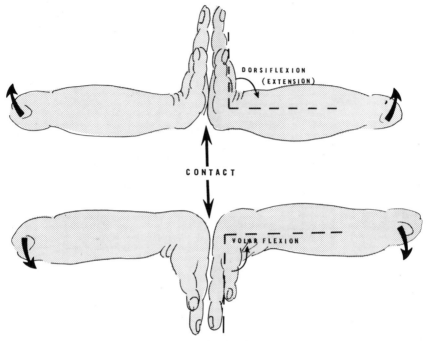

Figure 1–25. Clinical measurement of wrist flexion and extension. Wrist dorsiflexion (extension) can be estimated by placing the palms together and raising the elbows without allowing the palms to lose contact. Wrist palmar flexion can be determined by placing the backs of the hands together, finger facing down, and then lowering the elbows until the hands begin to separate.

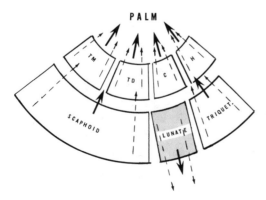

Figure 1–26. Carpal bone configuration, direction of displacement. The carpal bones by their shape form the palmar concavity and the dorsal concavity of the hand. The bones are broader on their dorsal surfaces and narrower on their palmar surface. This shape causes them to dislocate dorsally (with the exception of the lunate bone).

Since direct trauma to a carpal bone can cause widespread pain and impairment, identifying the precise location of the carpal bone involved can only be determined by a precise clinical examination. Palpation of the two styloids, the radial and ulnar, determines the forearm aspect of the wrist (see Fig. 1–11). There is usually a 14° obliquity of the radial-ulnar line (Figure 1–27).

The Navicular Bone. This bone, also known as the scaphoid bone, is the largest of the proximal row and is the most radial of proximal carpal bones. It is the floor of the "snuff box" (Fig. 1–28), which can be palpated. Ulnar deviation of the hand causes the navicular bone to slide out from under the overhanging radial styloid, so that it is directly palpable (Fig. 1–29). Except for the Colles' fracture of the radius, fracture of the navicular bone is the most common result of a fall upon the extended hand.

The location of the navicular can also be pinpointed by flexion of all the fingers. Lines drawn along the fingers and through the tips will converge on the navicular bone (Fig. 1–30).

Palpation of the Trapezium. The trapezium (also termed greater multangular) is located on the radial side of the hand, just distal to the navicular, and articulating with the first metacarpal. On deviating the hand in an ulnar direction, the trapezium can be palpated by shifting of the examiner's hand distally from the snuff box and the naivcular (Fig. 1–31). It is more easily palpated if the patient simultaneously flexes the thumb.

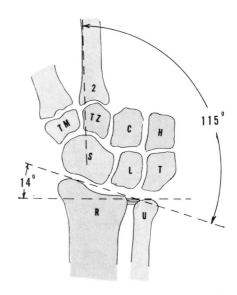

Figure 1–27. Normal alignment of carpal, radial, and metacarpal bones. The distal surface of the radius and ulna usually has an ulnar facing of 14°. The second metacarpal "fixed" to the trapezoid (TZ) is in direct alignment to the radius at a 115° angulation to the distal radial ulnar facing. R = radius; U = ulna; TM = trapezium;   S = sapphoid; L = lunate;   T = triquetrum;   2 = second metacarpal;   C = capitate; N = navicular.

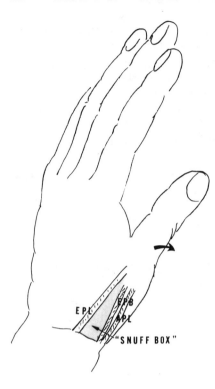

Figure 1-28. The "snuff box" is a palpable depression (shaded area) overlying the navicular bone. With the thumb abducted, the tendons of the extensor pollicis longus (EPL), the extensor pollicis brevis (EPB) and the abductor pollicis longus (APL) outline the depression of the box. In former generations snuff was placed there for inhalation, hence the term.

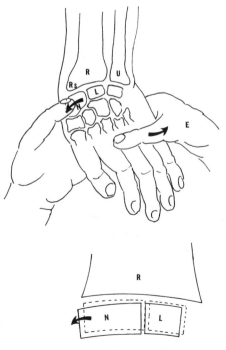

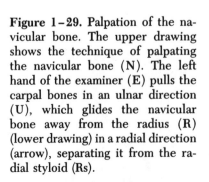

Figure 1-29. Palpation of the navicular bone. The upper drawing shows the technique of palpating the navicular bone (N). The left hand of the examiner (E) pulls the carpal bones in an ulnar direction (U), which glides the navicular bone away from the radius (R) (lower drawing) in a radial direction (arrow), separating it from the radial styloid (Rs).

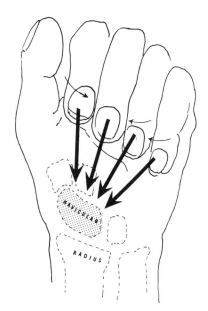

Figure 1–30. Direction of flexion immobilization in fractures of phalanges. The fingers normally flex across the palm in a direction towards the navicular (scaphoid) bone. The axis rotation about the middle finger (arrows) cannot be incorporated into casts or splints.

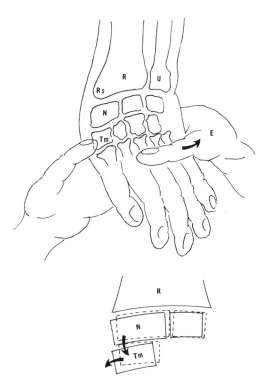

Figure 1–31. Palpation of the trapezium bone. The upper figure shows the technique of palpating the trapezium bone (Tm). The hand of the examiner (E) pulls the carpal row to the ulnar side (U), which glides the trapezium bone away from the navicular (N) bone in a radial direction (lower drawing), as shown by the curved arrows.

Palpation of the Trapezium–First Metacarpal Joint. Moving distally from the trapezium, with the hand deviated in an ulnar direction, the trapezium–first metacarpal articulation can be palpated (Fig. 1–32). Degenerative arthritic changes in the cartilage associated with this joint are commonly disabling and result from repetitive trauma to this circumferential articulation, which is used excessively in activities of daily living.

Palpation of Lister's Tubercle. Lister's tubercle, on the mid-dorsum of the radial head (Fig. 1–33), can be palpated as a landmark in determining the alignment of the lunate, capitate, and the third metacarpal bones.

Palpation of the Capitate Bone. From the alignment of Lister's tubercle to the third metacarpal bone, the capitate can be palpated. It lies in the distal carpal row, distal to the lunate bone and proximal to the head of the third metacarpal. The capitate bone has a central depression, which can be palpated when the hand is in a neutral position (upper drawing in Fig. 1–34); the depression is proximal to the head of the third metacarpal, which can also be palpated (lower drawing).

Palpation of the Lunate Bone. The lunate bone, just proximal to the capitate and aligned between Lister's tubercle and the third metacarpal bone, is clinically prominent. Because of its shape and alignment in the carpal row (Fig. 1–35), it is the most frequently dislocated and, after the navicular, the most commonly fractured carpal bone.

The lunate bone is palpable just proximal to the capitate and just distal to the radial tubercle. Clinically, with the patient's wrist flexed, the capitate bone can be palpated, and the examiner's finger can move proximally along the alignment towards Lister's tubercle (Fig. 1–36).

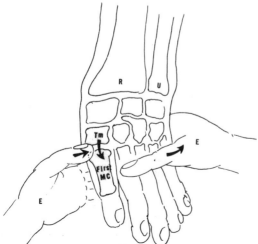

Figure 1–32. Palpation of the first metacarpal bone and the metacarpal-trapezium joint. The examiner's hand (right E) deviates the entire hand to the ulnar side (U), which opens the first metacarpal-trapezium joint and exposes the head of the first metacarpal bone to the examiner's other palpating hand (left E).

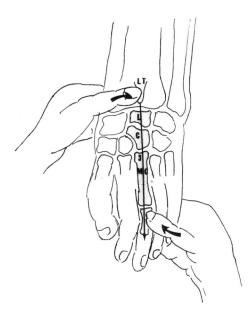

Figure 1–33. By placing the thumb on Lister's tubercle (LT) and holding the third finger, the examiner can determine the alignment of the lunate (L) and the capitate (C) with the radius.

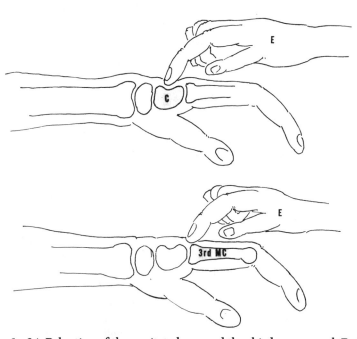

Figure 1–34. Palpation of the capitate bone and the third metacarpal. Realizing the alignment of the capitate to the Lister tubercle and the third metacarpal bone (see Fig. 1–33), the capitate can be palpated on the dorsum of the hand. It has a palpable depression on its dorsum. The base of the third metacarpal (lower picture) is palpated by moving distally from the capitate.

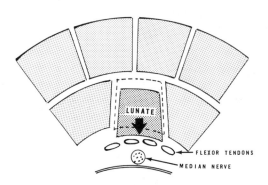

Figure 1–35. Dislocation of the lunate carpal bone. Except for the lunate, all the carpal bones dislocate dorsally because of their shape. From a fall upon the dorsiflexed hand, the lunate dislocates in a palmar direction, causing swelling on the volar surface of the wrist and compression of the flexor tendons of the fingers and median nerve.

The extensor carpi radialis brevis tendon lies over these bones, and attaches to the base of the third metacarpal.

The Triquetrum Bone. The triquetrum bone lies just distal to the ulnar styloid. To facilitate its palpation, the hand should be deviated in a radial direction, so as to move the triquetrum out from under the ulnar styloid (Fig. 1–37). The sesamoid bone lies directly over the triquetrum, with the result that palpation of this bone sometimes difficult. The triquetrum is vulnerable to injury and fracture.

The Pisiform Sesamoid Bone. The pisiform sesamoid bone is a ovoid bone within the flexor carpi ulnaris tendon and lies directly over the triquetrum (Fig. 1–38). It has a direct relationship to the proximal band of the transverse carpal ligament (Fig. 1–21).

The Hamate Bone. The hamate lies distal to the triquetrum bone in the distal carpal row. The hook of the hamate can be palpated directly below and inward from the pisiform bone (see Fig. 1–38).

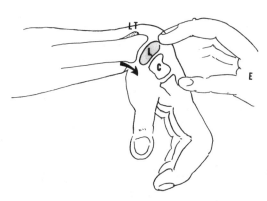

Figure 1–36. Palpation of the lunate bone. The lunate bone (L), located in the proximal carpal row, is in direct alignment with Lister's tubercle (LT), the capitate (C), and the third metacarpal bone. With the patient's wrist flexed (curved arrow), the examiner (E) can palpate the tubercle and the dorsal depression on the capitate and move slightly proximal along that line.

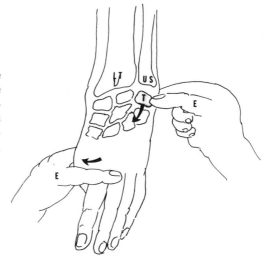

Figure 1–37. Palpation of the triquetrum. By deviating the patient's hand in a radial direction, the examiner causes the triquetrum (T) to move distally (curved arrow) from under the ulnar styloid (US), making it easier to palpate. Shown are the dorsum of the hand and the Lister tubercle (LT). The triquetrum is third highest in the number of carpal fractures.

Metacarpals

The four metacarpal bones articulate with the irregular border of the distal carpal row (Fig. 1–39). Examination of these metacarpals, starting at the radial side, begins with the first metacarpal, the thumb. The functional anatomy and thus the movements of the thumb are

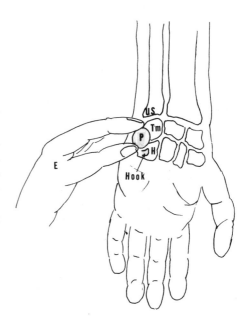

Figure 1–38. Palpation of the pisiform and the hook of the hamate. This palmar view of the hand depicts the site of the pisiform (sesamoid bone) distal to the ulnar styloid (US) and overlying the triquetrum (Tm). The examiner (E) can roll his thumb dorsally and radially and palpate the hook of the hamate bone (H), to which the tranverse carpal ligament is attached.

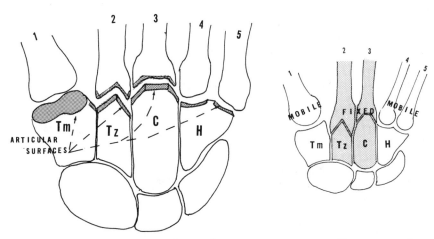

Figure 1–39. Carpometacarpal articulations. Five metacarpal bones articulate with four carpal bones. The second and the third metacarpals immobilize this segment by their numerous facets, close apposition of the planes of these facets, and the deep inset of the second metacarpal against the trapezoid and between the trapezium and the capitate. The first, fourth, and fifth metacarpals are mobile about this central fixed segment.

intricate, and demand definition (Fig. 1–40). The metacarpal moves upon a saddle-shaped (sellar) joint of the trapezium (Fig. 1–41) in a circumduction manner (Fig. 1–42). Opposition of the thumb is a combination of all motions: it begins as extension to abduction, proceeds into flexion, then into adduction. The muscles activating this motion will be subsequently discussed.

Palpation of the First Metacarpal. The first metacarpal is on the radial side of the hand; it is a continuation of the snuff box, which has been discussed and illustrated, and the trapezium bone (Fig. 1–43). Moving proximally, the joint between the base of the first metacarpal and the trapezium can be palpated, and its range can be noted by circumduction of the first metacarpal bone. This joint is a prominent site of symptomatic degenerative arthritic changes.

Palpation of the Second and Third Metacarpals. The second and third metacarpals form "immobile" joints. The second metacarpal has a gutter-shaped surface that fits over the central ridge of the trapezoid. The third metacarpal base has three opposing facets that fit directly into the three opposing facets of the capitate. These joints are "congruous" (close packed) and permit no motion.

These joints can be palpated by movement of the examiner's hand in an ulnar direction while the examiner's other hand stabilizes the carpal rows (Fig. 1–44).

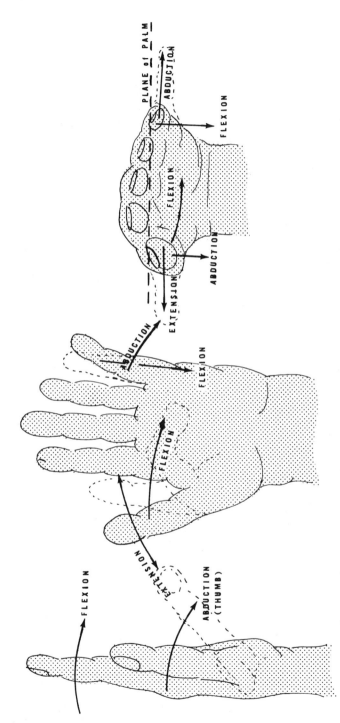

Figure 1–40. Definition of movement. Thumb: Extension consists of movement away from the radial side of the index finger in the plane of the palm. Abduction is movement away from the palm in a plan 90° to that of the plane of the palm. Flexion is made up of movement in a plane parallel to that of the palm so as to sweep the ulnar side of the thumb across the palm. Little finger: Extension involves full extension of all the joints of the little finger. Abduction consists of movement away from the ring finger in the plane of the palm. Flexion is 90° flexion of the finger at the metacarpophalangeal joints with the interphalangeal joints in extension.

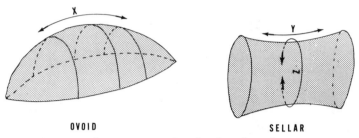

Figure 1–41. Joint surfaces are considered to be of two basic types: ovoid and sellar. Ovoid permits motion in one plane, X; sellar permits motion in two planes, Y and Z.

Palpation of the Fourth and Fifth Metacarpals. These two ulnar-placed metacarpals are mobile and articulate in a circumduction manner about the two concave facets of the hamate bone (Fig. 1 – 45). They essentially move about the central "fixed pillar" of the second and third metacarpals to "cup" the flexed hand.

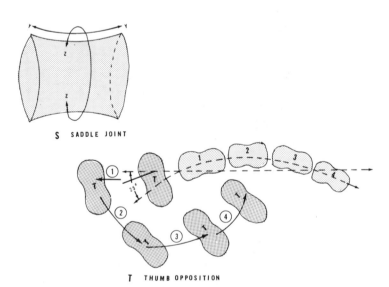

Figure 1–42. Thumb-metacarpal joint. The trapezium – first-metacarpal joint (thumb) is a saddle joint (S) in which two planes of motion that are tangential to each other are possible. The plane of the resting thumb (T) is 25° to the plane of the other metacarpals. Opposition of the thumb is a combination of consecutive motions: (1) extension in the plane of the palm, (2) into abduction into the palm, (3) flexion of the metacarpophalangeal joint, with (4) simultaneous adduction to the opposing finger.

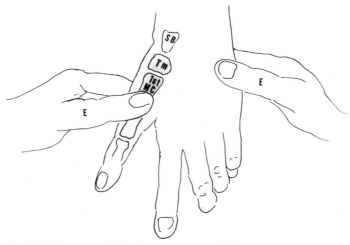

Figure 1–43. Palpation of the first metacarpal (thumb). Stabilizing the hand, the first metacarpal bone (1st MC), on the radial side of the hand distal to the trapezium (Tm) and the snuff box (SB), can be identified. Mobilization of this metacarpal tests the range of the metacarpal-carpal (1st MC and Tm) joint. This is a frequent site of degenerative joint disease.

When the hand is fully flexed, the distal ends of the metacarpal bones are palpable and a small groove is evident where the extensor tendons pass. The distal surface of the metacarpal is covered by hyaline cartilage that extends slightly over the dorsum and around the palmar surface on a rounded surface (Fig. 1–46).

Figure 1–44. Palpation of the immobile segment: the second and third metacarpals. Stabilizing the carpal rows with one hand, the second and third metacarpals (2nd MC and 3rd MC) can be mobilized against the facets of the trapezium (Tm) and the capitate (C). No significant movement is attainable at these joints.

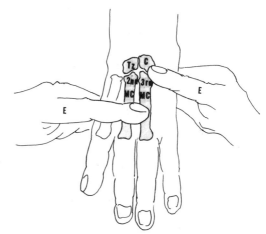

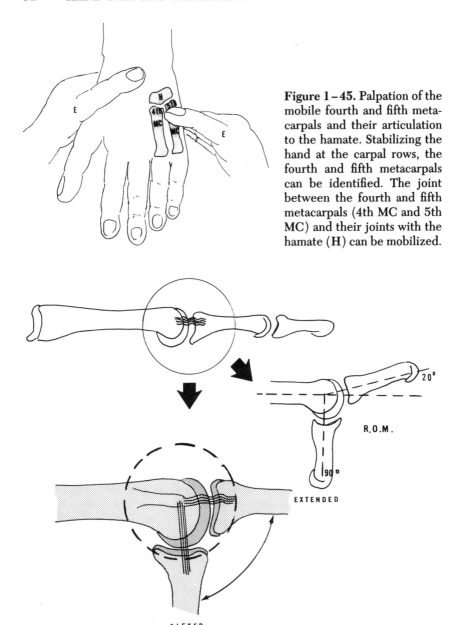

Figure 1–45. Palpation of the mobile fourth and fifth metacarpals and their articulation to the hamate. Stabilizing the hand at the carpal rows, the fourth and fifth metacarpals can be identified. The joint between the fourth and fifth metacarpals (4th MC and 5th MC) and their joints with the hamate (H) can be mobilized.

Figure 1–46. Metacarpophalangeal joints. As a result of the eccentric radius of rotation about the axis of the head of the metacarpal (dotted circle), flexion of the phalanx causes the collateral ligaments to become taut. The laxity of the ligaments is extension permits some lateral motion. Range of motion (ROM) is 90° flexion and 20° hyperextension. Darker shading on the ends of the bones indicates cartilage.

Abduction and adduction of the metacarpophalangeal joint is limited when the finger is flexed because the head is flattened at its distal margin and the collateral ligaments are taut in flexion. The collateral ligaments originate from a small tubercle eccentrically located on the lateral surfaces of the head. With the finger extended, the ligaments are slack, permitting lateral movement. In the flexed position, the base of the phalanx seats firmly against the metacarpal head because of its ovoid shape (Fig. 1 – 47). In flexion, therefore, the ligament becomes taut. On the palmar aspect, the condyles are broader than on the dorsal aspect, further tightening the collateral ligaments.

There are no ligaments on the dorsal surface of the metacarpophalangeal joints to limit motion. Any limitation is imposed by fibrocartilaginous "palmar plates" (Fig. 1 – 48). The distal portion is cartilaginous and firmly attached to the proximal portion of the phalanx. The proximal portion of the plate is membranous and is loosely attached to the metacarpal. The looser connection makes this portion of the plate prone to separation from its attachment in the event of a subluxation. Prolonged immobilization of a finger in the flexed position can cause retraction of the membranous portion of the plate and result in a joint "flexion contracture."

The plates reinforce the joint capsules and are interposed between the joints and the flexor tendons that traverse the joint. They are firmly held against the joints by fibers of the collateral ligaments, and are connected by deep transverse ligaments (Fig. 1 – 49). These intermetacarpal ligaments have an outpouching on the palmar surfaces, termed the "vaginal ligament," which encloses the flexor tendons. These pouches form part of the lubricating apparatus of the flexor tendons and prevent bowing.

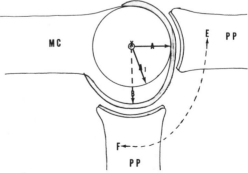

Figure 1–47. Incongruity of the metacarpal-proximal phalangeal joint. Were the head of the metacarpal bone a perfect circle (A), the proximal phalanx (PP) would flex (F) extend (E) in perfect rotation. The head of the metacarpal is ovoid, however, with the palmar edge (B) being further from the axis (X); thus flexion (F) and extension (E) of the proximal phalanx traces an eliptical curve (dotted line). The collateral ligaments going from the axis of rotation (X) are slack in phalanx extension and taut in phalanx flexion, as the distance increases from A to B.

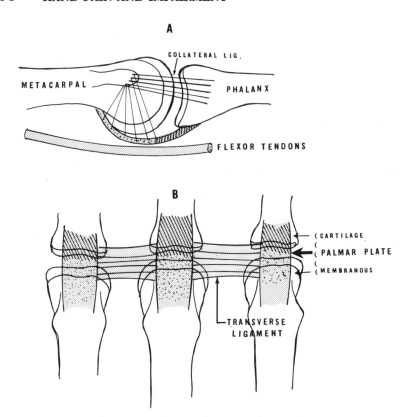

Figure 1–48. Palmar plate. A fibrocartilaginous plate replaces the ligament on the palmar surface of the joint. The plate is firmly held to the metacarpal by fibers of the collateral ligament. (*A*) The cartilaginous portion is firmly attached to the phalanx. (*B*) Palmar view shows the deep transverse ligament that connects the plates and prevents lateral motion of all the metacarpals except the thumb. The proximal membranous portion is loosely attached to the metacarpal.

PHALANGES

There are 14 phalanges in each hand. The thumb has two, and the other four fingers, three each. Joint terminology indicates that the distal end of the proximal phalanx articulates upon the proximal surface of the middle phalanx, forming the proximal interphalangeal (PIP) joint. The distal end of the middle phalanx articulates with the proximal surface of the distal phalanx, forming the distal interphalangeal (DIP) joint (Fig. 1–50).

The interphalangeal joints are true hinge joints, allowing only flexion and extension (Fig. 1–51). In comparison, the metacarpophalangeal joints:

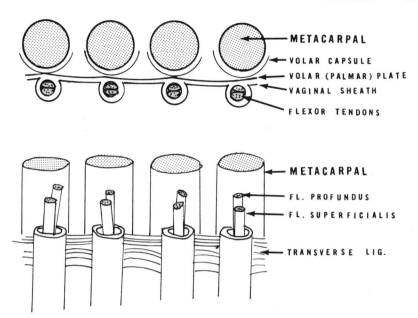

- METACARPAL
- VOLAR CAPSULE
- VOLAR (PALMAR) PLATE
- VAGINAL SHEATH
- FLEXOR TENDONS

- METACARPAL
- FL. PROFUNDUS
- FL. SUPERFICIALIS
- TRANSVERSE LIG.

Figure 1–49. Transverse metacarpal ligament. The volar fibrocartilaginous plate reinforces the joint capsule. It also forms the dorsal portion of the vaginal ligament that forms pouches that encircle the flexor tendons as part of the tendons' gliding mechanism.

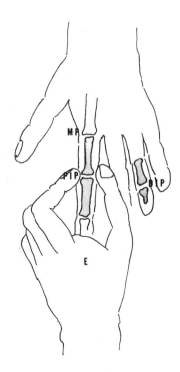

Figure 1–50. Palpation of the joints of the fingers. The metacarpal joint (MP) can be palpated by the examiner (E), as can the proximal interphalangeal joint (PIP) and the distal interphalangeal joint (DIP).

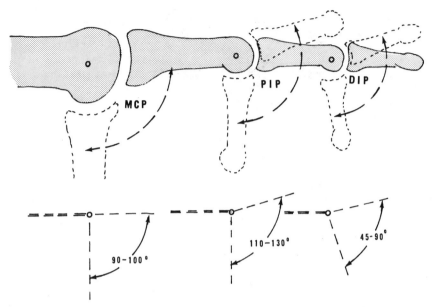

Figure 1–51. Range of motion of the interphalangeal joints. The proximal interphalangeal joint (PIP) averages 110° to 130° and the distal interphalangeal joints (DIP), 45° to 90°. Both of these joints are capable of hyperextension. Further flexion is checked by the dorsal capsule. The metacarpophalangeal joint (MCP) has a range of 90° to 100°.

1. Permit abduction, adduction, and circumduction (being ball-and-socket joints).
2. Have structural articular configurations as noted.
3. Permit passive hyperextension (Fig. 1–52), which is not possible at the interphalangeal joint.
4. Have collateral ligaments that are slack in the extended position and taut in flexion, whereas the interphalangeal joints do not.
5. Have palmar plates at the metacarpophalangeal joints that, with their attachments (deep transverse ligament, interossei tendons, and palmar aponeurosis), permit a flexibility not available to the interphalangeal joints.

MUSCULAR CONTROL OF THE HAND

The passive examination of the hand, its bones and joints, may now be extended to regarding its neuromuscular control. This can be considered an "active" examination, since the patient's cooperation is man-

Figure 1–52. Grades of extension range of motion of the metacarpophalangeal joint. As passive extension is possible at the metacarpophalangeal joint to a larger degree than at other finger joints, an arbitrary degree system has been postulated. Normally Grade 1 (45° extension) is considered physiological and greater degrees of extension are considered hyperextension.

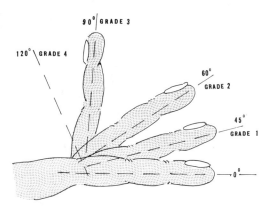

dated. Neuromuscular control implies mental capability, the proper neurological control system (to be discussed in Chapter 2), and adequate tendon action (to be discussed in Chapter 4).

Muscular control of the hand implicates forearm muscles and extrinsic and intrinsic hand muscle groups.

Extrinsic Muscles

All forearm muscles motorizing the hand traverse the wrist joint and the metacarpal joints. The palmar group originates from the medial condyle of the humerus and is flexor in function. The dorsal group originates from the lateral condyle of the humerus and is essentially extensor in function.

The dorsal group of extensor forearm muscles (Fig. 1–53) is composed of superficial and deep layers, with the superficial layer divided into lateral and posterior groups. The lateral and posterior groups of the superficial layer are separated by the intrinsic muscles of the thumb (see Fig. 1–53).

The superficial group originates from the common extensor tendon, which is attached to the lateral epicondylar area, the intermuscular septum, and the lateral supracondylar ridge (Fig. 1–54).

I. Superficial extensor muscles
    A. Lateral group
        1. Brachioradialis. Not a hand muscle, it crosses the cubital fossa, inserts into the base of the styloid process of the radius, and flexes the elbow when the forearm is midway between pronation and supination.

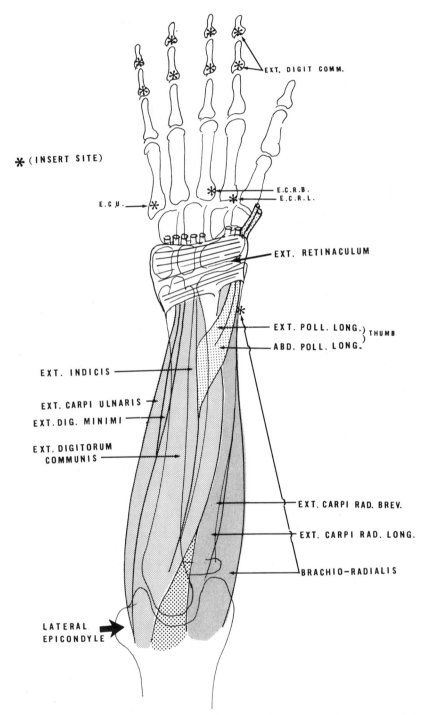

Figure 1–53. Extensor muscles of the forearm. The origin and insertion of the extensor muscles are shown as viewed in the left arm and hand. The extensor groups comprise superficial and deep layers which are divided by the extrinsic thumb muscles.

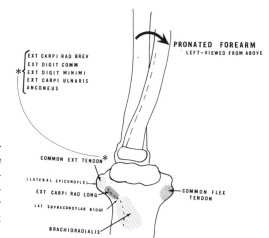

Figure 1-54. Origin of muscles about the elbow. The common extensor tendon originates from the lateral humeral epicondyle. the view presented is the pronated left elbow seen from above.

2. Extensor carpi radialis longus. Originating from the supracondylar ridge, it inserts into the base of the second metacarpal and activates the wrist.
3. Extensor carpi radialis brevis. Originating from the common tendon, it crosses the snuff box with the extensor carpi radialis longus, and inserts into the base of the middle metacarpal. It is also a pure wrist extensor.

B. Posterior group
1. Extensor indicis, extensor digitorum communis, extensor digiti minimi and extensor carpi ulnaris. These originate from the common extensor tendon. All, except the extensor carpi ulnaris, which insets into the base of the fifth metacarpal and extends the wrist, extend aspects of the digits that will be discussed.
2. Anconeus. It does not affect the fingers or wrist. It originates from the lateral epicondyle and crosses obliquely to insert into the posterior surface of the ulna.

II. Deep layer of the forearm extensors
A. Supinator. It does not affect the wrist or fingers, but supinates the forearm.
B. Abductor pollicis longus. It abducts the thumb.
C. Extensor pollicis brevis and extensor pollicis longus. Arising from the midregion of the ulna and radius and the interosseous membrane between them, they proceed obliquely "over" the wrist extensors and attach to the thumb and index fingers.

The Palmar Flexor Muscles. These originate from the medial condylar area of the humerus (Fig. 1–55) and are divided into two groups: the "superficial" and "deep."

I. Superficial group—originates as a common muscle mass from the medial epicondylar region.
   A. Pronator quadratus. Extending from the ridge of the ulna to insert upon the anterior surface of the radius, it acts merely upon the forearm.
   B. Flexor carpi radialis. Inserting upon the bases of the second and third metacarpals, it activates only the wrist.
   C. Palmaris longus: It acts only upon the wrist and is missing in 15 percent of the population.
   D. Flexor carpi ulnaris. Attaching to the pisiform sesamoid and the fifth metacarpal bones, it acts to flex the wrist toward the ulna, dividing into two heads, through which passes the ulnar nerve.

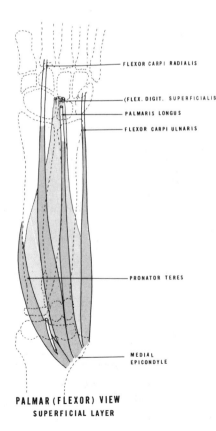

FLEXOR CARPI RADIALIS

(FLEX. DIGIT. SUPERFICIALIS

PALMARIS LONGUS

FLEXOR CARPI ULNARIS

PRONATOR TERES

MEDIAL
EPICONDYLE

PALMAR (FLEXOR) VIEW
SUPERFICIAL LAYER

Figure 1–55. Palmar flexor group, superficial layer. The superficial group of flexor muscles on the palmar surface of the forearm originate from a common muscle mass at the medial epicondyle. The most medial is the pronator teres, followed by the flexor carpi radialis inserting into the base of the second and third metacarpals, the palmaris longus, and the flexor carpi ulnaris attaching to the pisiform. The flexor digitorum in the deeper layer is seen through the superficial layer.

II. Deep layer—originates from sites on the palmar aspect of the radius and ulna (Fig. 1–56).

A. Sublimis. It originates from the medial condyle, coronoid processes of the ulna, and palmar surface of the radius. It ends in four tendons that insert into the bases of the second, third, fourth, and fifth middle phalanges. The sublimis separates into two portions.

1. Superficial (two tendons to the middle and ring fingers).

2. Deep (two tendons to the index and little fingers).

B. Profundus. It arises from the ulna and the interosseous membrane, crosses the wrist under the carpal ligament (Fig. 1–57) within the carpal tunnel, and attaches to the distal phalanges after perforating the sublimis (superficial) tendons (Fig. 1–58).

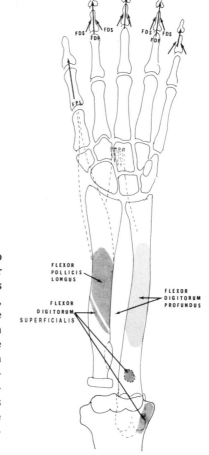

Figure 1–56. Palmar flexor group, deep layer. The deep layer contains the finger flexors. The flexor digitorum superficialis originates from the medial epicondyle, the coronoid process of the ulna, and the palmar surface of the radius. It ends in four tendons attached to the base of the middle phalanges. The flexor digitorum profundus arises from the ulna and interosseous membrane and insets into the distal phalanges. The flexor pollicis longus originates from the palmar surface of the radius and inserts into the base of the distal phalanx of the thumb.

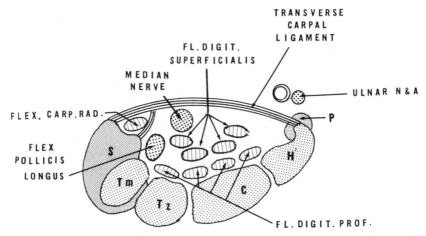

Figure 1-57. Contents of the carpal tunnel. The concave palmar surface of the carpal rows is crossed by the transverse carpal ligament. The tunnel contains the median nerve and all the flexor tendons and their sheaths. Thickening of the tendon sheaths, the carpal ligament, or deformation of the bony structure can compress the median nerve.

The previous discussion of muscles in the standard manner outlined their origin and insertion, which are confusing. Lampe[5] in 1951 proposed a "functional" terminology that is more practical and meaningful. He proposed naming muscles for their function not their location.

It would better serve the ultimate purpose of functional anatomy if

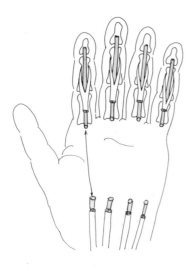

Figure 1-58. Insertion of flexor tendons. At the wrist the flexor sublimis tendons are arranged in two layers—the two inner tendons lying deep, and the two outer more superficially. In their course these tendons split to allow the profundus tendons to pass through then attach to the middle phalanges of the four medial fingers. The flexor profundus tendons at the the wrist are in one layer and in the same sheath as the sublimis. They pass between the split of the sublimis tendons to attach to the base of the distal phalanges.

the palmar group (flexor carpi radialis and ulnaris, flexor digitorum sublimis and profundus, pronator teres, and quadratus) were termed the "flexor pronator group." The dorsal group (extensor carpi radialis longus and brevis, extensor digitorum communis, indicis proprius, digiti quinti proprius, extensor pollicis brevis and longus, abductor pollicis longus, and supinator) would be termed "extensor assistant supinator." A thought could be given to further dividing the functional terminology to separate the forearm-wrist from the fingers.[6]

The nerve supply, an examination of which comprises the entire second chapter, could also be better described in functional terms. The radial nerve could be termed the "extensor assistant supinator nerve," the ulnar nerve termed the "finger spreader approximator nerve," and the median nerve the "flexor pronator thumb-finger approximator nerve." These terms, allegedly unwieldly, are functionally practical and meritorious of further thought and definition.

Tendinous Insertion into the Digits

Flexor Tendons. Each profundus tendon inserts into the base of the distal phalanx (see Fig. 1–58). It is cylindrical, but flattens as it passes the divided superficialis tendon where it flattens from front to back.

The superficialis tendon divides at the midpoint off the proximal phalanx (Fig. 1–59). Over the proximal middle phalanx articulation, it divides into a medial and lateral extension to form a "V." Each extension in turn divides and crosses over to the opposite side (see Fig. 1–59). The final division, a quarter of the original tendon (half of the split) passes "under" the profundus tendon, which has passed through the perforation (initial division) of the superficialis tendon.

Each flexor tendon is enveloped within a tubular sheath (Fig. 1–60) that contains a lubricating fluid similar to synovial fluid. These sheaths and their fluid diminish friction of the moving tendons at their points of angulation and curvature.

There are similar sheaths, termed bursae, protecting the flexor tendons in the palm. These sheaths are compartments (tunnels) related to the palmar fascia (Fig. 1–61) The palmar fascia (aponeurosis) crosses the palm (Fig. 1–62) forming fibrous compartments (tunnels) for the flexor tendons (Fig. 1–63). As the palmar fascia passes distally from the transverse carpal ligament, it divides into four bands that pass down to the four metacarpals. When the fascia reaches the metacarpal heads, it blends with the deep transverse ligament. The tendons of the profundus and superficialis are contained within these compartments.

The length of the extrinsic finger muscle tendons does not permit isolated motion of the fingers without simultaneous coordinated wrist action. It is not possible to fully extend the wrist and fingers together, as the flexors (profundus and superficialis) are not long enough to permit further extension.

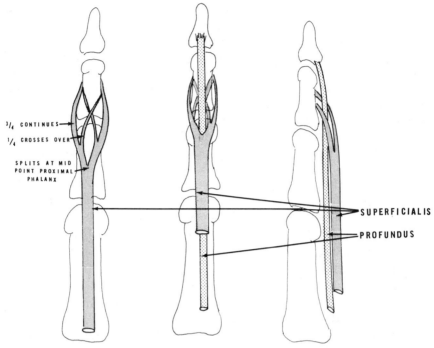

Figure 1–59. Digital flexor mechanism. The profundus tendon inserts into the entire breadth of the base of the distal phalanx, into the palmar plate, into the pulp of the finger. The superficialis tendon splits midway past the proximal phalanx. Three fourths of the fibers continue and attach to the lateral crest of the middle phalanx. One fourth crosses under the tendon of the profundus which has passed through the perforation of the superficialis tendon.

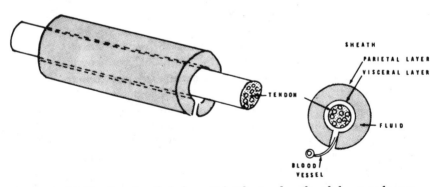

Figure 1–60. Tendon sheath (schematic). The tendon sheath has two layers— the parietal and the visceral, between which is a synovial fluid that acts as a lubricant. The blood vessel supplying the tendon enters by way of a fold in the sheath.

Figure 1–61. Tendon sheaths and flexor bursa. The tendon sheaths of the index, middle, and ring fingers extend from the midpalmar crease to the insertion of the flexor profundus tendon into the distal phalanx. The sheath of the fifth finger continues from the ulnar bursa which is found in the palm under the transverse carpal ligament. This bursa contains all the tendons except the thumb tendon. The ulnar bursa forms three compartments— one superficial to the sublimis tendons, one between the sublimis and profundus tendons, and one under the profundus tendons. The thumb bursa (radial bursa) extends from under the transverse carpal ligament to accompany the flexor tendon to its insertion at the distal phalanx. In 15%–20% of persons, the fifth tendon sheath does not communicate with the ulnar bursa. Occasionally all tendon sheaths connect with the bursa.

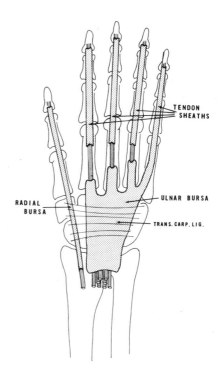

Tenodesis action is required. The term tenodesis[2] denotes "Surgical fixation of a tendon in order to restore muscle balance. . . or . . . to increase active power of joint motion." It should be a functional term indicating neuromuscular action to insure maximum functional action. In the hand, maximum finger flexion action occurs when the wrist is extended. With the wrist flexed, finger flexion strength is diminished.

Reciprocal relaxation of the extensors is necessary for adequate flexion. This is neurologically assured.[7,8] There is also a "lengthening" (viscoelastic) process of the tissues involved, in which deceleration is implemented. The extensors undergo viscoelastic decelerating elongation as the flexors contract, along with neurological reciprocal relaxation (Fig. 1–64).

Intrinsic Muscles

As discussed, the extrinsic muscles originate outside the hand. The intrinsic muscles originate within the hand and act upon the digits. They comprise the following groups:

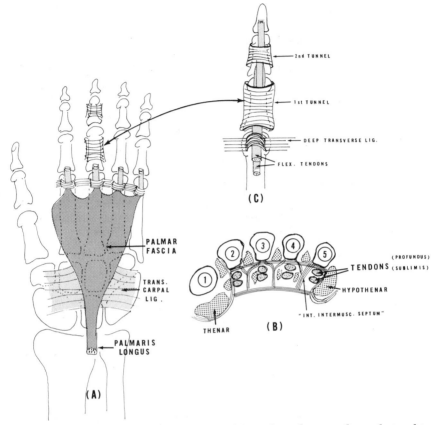

Figure 1–62. Palmar fascia. The course of the palmar fascia and its relationship to the tendons and transverse ligaments at the metacarpophalangeal joints are shown. (A) Passage of the palmar fascia over the transverse carpal ligament and fanning out to the four medial fingers. (B) The septa arising from the fascia and descending to the metacarpals to form compartments, each containing the flexor tendons and the intrinsic muscles. (C) The fibrous tunnels that enclose the flexor tendons during their passage along the phalanges.

1. The thenar group: performing thumb functions.
2. The hypothenar group: performing little (fifth) finger function.
3. The interossei and lumbricals: performing abduction and adduction of the fingers. They also combine with the extensor tendons to extend the fingers.

The interossei and the lumbrical muscles have a similar function, although the interossei are more consistently present and are stronger than the lumbricals.

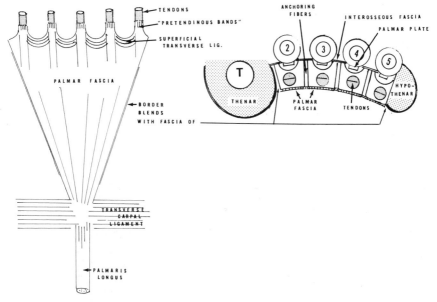

Figure 1–63. Palmar fascia (schematic). This is the triangular layer of fascia with its apex continuous with the transverse carpal ligament. It often unites with the palmaris longus. Distally it fans out over the heads of the metacarpals into thickened pretendinous bands that overlie the flexor tendons. Transverse fibers unite these bands forming the superficial transverse ligament. The lateral border of the palmer fascia blends with the fascia of the thenar and hypothenar muscle groups. Fibrous bands proceed dorsally to the interosseous fascia between the metacarpals forming compartments for the flexor tendons. The most medial (ulnar) layer is thick and is termed the internal intermuscular septum. The deep transverse metacarpal ligament blends with the flexor palmar plates (see Fig. 1–62) and forms fibrous sheaths into tunnels. Fibrous sheaths extend from the palmar fascia distally to the distal phalanx near the insertion of the profundus tendon. The deep transverse metacarpal ligament forms two tunnels which become thin at the joints to permit flexibility.

The interossei are supplied by the ulnar nerve and consist of four dorsal (Fig. 1–65) and three palmar muscles. The dorsal interossei are bipenniform muscles that arise from adjacent sides of the opposing metacarpals and converge into lateral bands that attach to the extensor mechanism. The first dorsal interosseous muscle originates from two bellies, inserts upon the radial side of the first metacarpal, and produces *ad*duction of this metacarpal. It always inserts upon bone. The radial artery passes between the two heads of this muscle's origin.

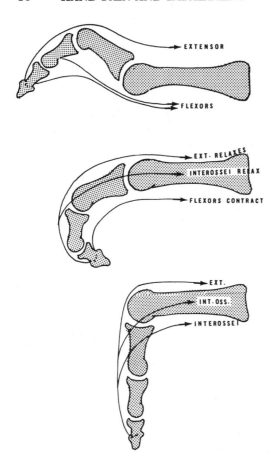

EXTENSOR

FLEXORS

EXT. RELAXES

INTEROSSEI RELAX

FLEXORS CONTRACT

EXT.

INT. OSS.

INTEROSSEI

Figure 1–64. Full flexion of the digits. Normally there is action of both extensors and flexors during finger flexion. Pure action of the flexors and extensors will cause a clawing, therefore, during flexion the extensors relax their viscoelastic property as do the intrinsics (interossei). The interossei flex the metacarpophalangeal joint when the interphalangeal joints are extended.

The second and third interossei insert upon the middle finger, and the fourth inserts upon the ulnar side of the ring finger. Their function is *ab*duction of the index and ring fingers from the midline; they may move the middle finger in either a medial or lateral direction. In half the population, these muscles attach upon bone, and in the rest, they are attached to the extensor mechanism. The interosseus tendons pass dorsally to the transverse palmar ligament (Fig. 1–66). The three palmar interosseous muscles (Fig. 1–67) function as *ad*ductors of the fingers toward the middle finger. The first palmar interosseous arises from the ulnar side of the second metacarpal and attaches to the extensor mechanism on the same side of the metacarpal. The second interosseus originates from the radial side of the fourth metacarpal, and the third from the little (fifth) finger to attach to the extensor mechanism on the radial side.

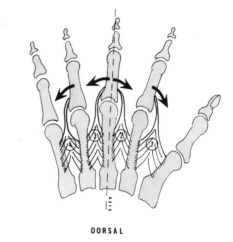

DORSAL

Figure 1–65. Dorsal interossei muscles. The dorsal interossei muscles with the abductor pollicis to the thumb and the abductor digiti quinti spread the fingers, that is, move them away from the axial line of the hand. The interossei arise from double muscle bellies. They pass dorsally to the transverse palmar ligaments. The first interosseus usually attaches to the bone and the others to the extensor tendon expansion.

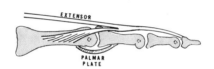

Figure 1–66. Relationship of intrinsics to the transverse ligament. The figure to the left is the palmar view of the left hand. The lumbrical originates from the flexor tendon passing dorsally to the ultimate union with the interossei into the extensor mechanism.

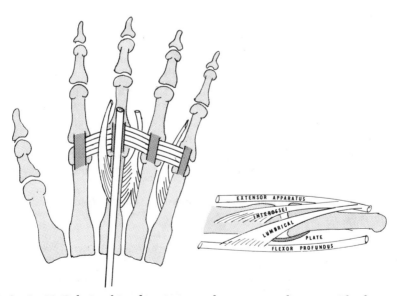

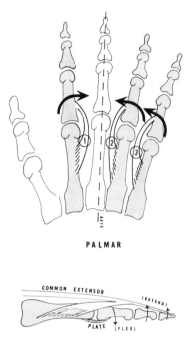

PALMAR

COMMON EXTENSOR

(EXTEND)

PLATE (FLEX)

Figure 1–67. Palmar interossei, finger adductors. The thumb has its own adductor. There are only three palmar interossei arising from the second, fourth, and fifth metacarpals. The tendons pass dorsally to attach to the common extensor tendons. They adduct the fingers, flex the metacarpophalangeal joint, and extend the proximal interphalangeal joints.

There are (usually) four lumbrical muscles (see Fig. 1–66). They arise from the radial side of the tendons of the flexor digitorum profundus and pass along the same side of the corresponding finger to attach to the extensor mechanism. Whereas the seven interossei pass "behind" the deep transverse ligament, the lumbricals pass in front of the ligament. They are accompanied by the digital nerves. The function of the lumbricals is to confer precision rather than strength. Long found no lumbrical activity in the power grip,[9] and the lumbricals are richly innervated with sensory nerve endings, which may conceivably elicit proprioception and ensure balance between flexion and extension in precision finger activities.

The mode of operation of the interosseous and other muscles could be clarified by using functional terminology. Thus,

1. The interossei could be termed "muscles lying on each side of the finger," rather than "dorsal" and "palmar."
2. The first dorsal interosseus would become the "flexor-radial deviator" and "rotator" of the first metacarpal joint.
3. The first dorsal interosseus would also become an "extensor of the two distal phalanges of the middle finger."
4. The interossei of the other fingers would "flex" and "rotate" these fingers.

5. The interossei of the second, third, and fourth fingers would also "extend" the distal two digits.
6. The lumbricals would be described an "interphalangeal extensors."

Clinical examination of the interossei and lumbricals is done by carrying out functional movements involving the "hook grip," the "power grip" (Fig. 1–68), and the hammer position. The latter requires a firm grip; the fingers flex in a marked "ulnar" deviation; and rotation brings them into opposition with the thenar eminence. The wrist also deviates in an ulnar deviation to bring the hammer handle in alignment with the forearm. This wrist action must be correlated with finger action, and must be proprioceptively coordinated.

When precision, not force is required the lumbricals are utilized. Pure anatomic finger flexion produces opposition of the thumb tip to the index side, whereas precise tip-to-tip opposition requires rotation and ulnar deviation of the index finger. (Fig. 1–69). These motions,

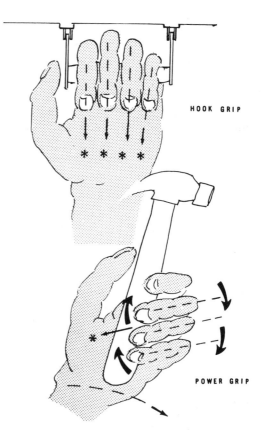

HOOK GRIP

POWER GRIP

Figure 1–68. Motion of fingers in functional movements. The hook grip is used rarely but functions to hold or lift luggage or in turning a key when the thumb presses against the side of the middle phalanx on the index finger. In the power grip, used when hammering, the fingers are flexed and rotated in ulnar deviation. The fingers flex towards the thenar eminence. The wrist also moves in an ulnar deviation, placing the hammer in alignment with the forearm. The hand grips and the wrist moves the hammer.

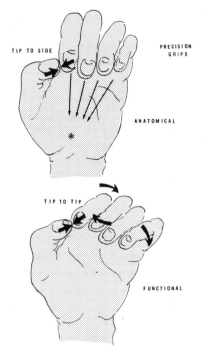

Figure 1-69. Motion of fingers in functional movements. The precision grip requires finger tip-to-tip approximation. If pure finger flexion is used, the fingers flex towards the palm causing the thumb to first finger approximation to be tip-to-side. To cause tip-to-tip approximation, the fingers must rotate and deviate in an ulnar direction.

utilizing rotation and ulnar deviation, are proprioceptively controlled through the coordinated action of the interossei upon the proximal phalanges and the richly innervated lumbricals. The precise kinesiology of finger function has been clarified by electromyographic studies.[10,11]

The abductors of the fingers are clinically evaluated by manually resisting the spread of all the fingers (Fig. 1-70).

Phalanges

Extensor Digital Mechanisms. The four tendons of the extensor digitorum pass over the dorsum of the hand and under the extensor retinaculum at the wrist, where they are enclosed within a synovial sheath (Fig. 1-71). From there they proceed along the dorsum of the phalanges.

The extensor tendon splits at the distal end of the proximal phalanx, where it becomes joined with the intrinsic musculature (lumbricals and interossei) to form the "extensor apparatus" of the finger (Fig. 1-72). Each lateral band is joined by half of an interosseous muscle tendon. More distally, each is joined by the lumbrical tendon, the union being located upon the dorsum of the proximal phalanx. These combined tendons ultimately attach to the middle and distal phalanges in conjunction with the lateral bands of the extensor expansion. The course and

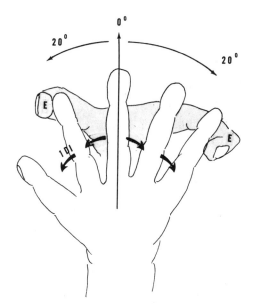

Figure 1–70. Clinical examination of the intrinsic abductors of the hand. With the middle finger (0°) as the "fixed" base the index finger and the fourth and fifth fingers abduct to approximately 20° in each direction. The examiner (**E**) determines the strength and the range of motion.

points of attachments of the extensor mechanism are schematically depicted in Fig. 1–73).

Without the combined action of the intrinsics, "pure" extensor digitorum action would extend the metacarpophalangeal joint and "flex" the interphalangeal joints (see A in Fig. 1–74) due to active pull of the extensors and passive pull of the flexor digitorum profundus.

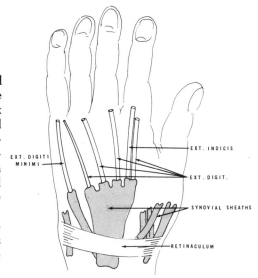

Figure 1–71. Dorsum of hand showing tendon sheaths of the extensor tendons. There are six fibro-osseous tunnels (synovial sheaths) passing under the extensor retinaculum. The extensor indicis enters the common sheath to proceed to the medial aspect of the first finger, there joining the extensor tendon. The extensor digiti quinti (proprius) has its own sheath. It is the major extensor of the little finger.

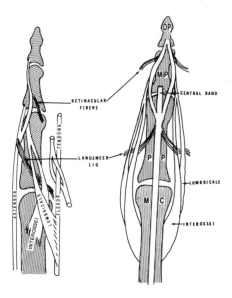

Figure 1–72. Extensor apparatus of the fingers. The extensor communis tendon divides into three components at the distal end of the proximal phalanx—a central and two lateral bands. The central band inserts into the proximal end of the middle phalanx (MP). The lateral bands pass over the lateral aspects of the proximal interphalangeal joints to converge over the middle phalanx and insert into the proximal portion of the distal phalanx (DP). A thin layer of fascia extends laterally from the extensor tendon forming a hood that encircles the interossei and lumbrical muscles (Figs. 1–78 and 1–79).

Extension of the fingers requires combined action of the long extensors and the intrinsics. Extension of the proximal interphalangeal joint occurs because of the combined action of three elements. The central band of the extensor tendon inserts into the base of the middle phalanx; the two lateral bands pass to either side of the proximal interphalangeal joint to fuse distally on the mid-dorsum of the middle phalanx, and ultimately insert into the distal phalanx.

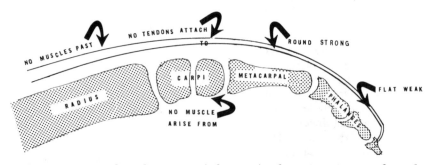

Figure 1–73. Dorsal tendon course (schematic). The course, points of attachment, and areas of attachment of the extensor tendons on the dorsum of the hand and fingers are shown.

Figure 1–74. Combined action of the long extensors and intrinsics. (*A*) Pure extensor tendon pull (without intrinsics) extends the metacarpophalangeal and flexes the proximal interphalangeal joints owing to *passive* pull of the flexors on the distal phalanges. (*X*) As the extensor contracts, the F_{fdp} (flexor) relaxes. The interossei F_1

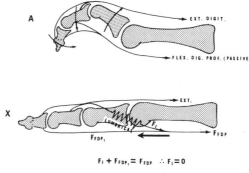

$$F_1 + F_{FDP_1} = F_{FDP} \quad \therefore F_1 = 0$$

contracts drawing the flexor tendon forward to decrease the passive pull of the flexors. $F_1 = 0$ indicates *no flexion* force at the metacarpophalangeal joint. Three muscular actions are required to extend the fingers—(1) extensor digitorum longus, (2) passive profundus, and (3) lumbrical pull upon the flexor tendon in a distal direction to relax the passive pull.

The middle phalanx extends by virtue of the central slip, whereas the distal phalanx extends by the two combined slips. The length of these slips must be in proper balance to effectively extend the finger. In the case of injury or disease, proper surgical reconstruction requires that this balance be achieved to ensure proper function.

Retinacular Ligaments. There are two groups of fibers that form the extensive retinacular system of the hand: the dorsal and the lateral retinacular system. Landsmeer analyzed the anatomy and function of these fibers and gave them their name "retinacular ligaments."[12]

Each ligament is formed by a lateral lamina, a longitudinal cord, and oblique cutaneous fibers. The lateral lamina has transverse and oblique fibers that cover the collateral ligaments of the proximal interphalangeal joint (Fig. 1–75). They are transverse in their proximal part and oblique in their distal part.

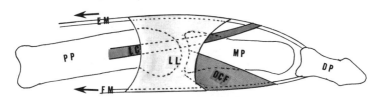

Figure 1–75. Retinacular ligaments. The lateral lamina (LL), the oblique cutaneous fibers (OBF) and the longitudinal cord (LC) connect the extensor mechanism (EM) and the flexor mechanism (FM) as they control motion of the proximal phalanx (PP), the middle phalanx (MP) and the distal phalanx (DP). See text for precise function.

The longitudinal cord is thick and comprised of few fibers. It runs under the lateral lamina, initially running dorsally to the joint over which it resides. The oblique cutaneous fibers run obliquely from a bony insertion of the neck of the proximal phalanx to attach to the dermis at the middle phalanx.

Allegedly the lateral lamina of the retinacular ligaments becomes tense during finger extension and flexion so as to maintain the isometrics of the extensor mechanism. The longitudinal cord also contributes to the stability and conjoined movements of the fingers, and the oblique cutaneous fibers stabilize the palmar skin during finger actions.

There have been conflicts over the precise function of the retinacular ligaments.[13] Their role in extending the digit[14] has been questioned, but since the lateral lamina becomes taut during finger extension it possibly limits and "maintains isometrics of the extensor mechanism,"[13] (Fig. 1–76) and the longitudinal cord contributes to the stability of the proximal interphalangeal joint. The oblique cutaneous fibers probably stabilize the palmar skin during finger prehension.

The lateral bands of the extensor mechanism migrate dorsally as the proximal interphalangeal joint extends (Fig. 1–77). This is permitted by the elasticity of the triangular ligament.

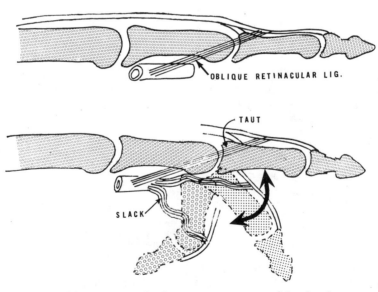

Figure 1–76. Oblique retinacular ligament. Extension of the distal joint is aided by the tenodesis action of the retinacular ligament as the proximal joint extends. In the flexed position, the ligament is slack.

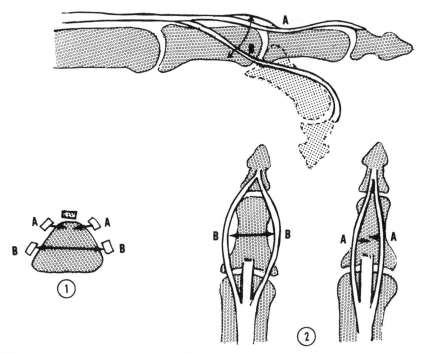

Figure 1–77. Dorsal migration of extensor lateral bands. With full extension being due to the shape of the phalanx (1), and the bands becoming taut (upper figure, (A), on the dorsum the bands extend approximately from (A) to (A). In (2), the left figure is the flexed phalanx, and the right figure the extended phalanx. The lateral bands migrate dorsally as the proximal interphalangeal joint extends. This is permitted by the elastic quality of the triangular ligament.

At the distal end of the metacarpal, the extensor tendon flattens to resemble fascia and wraps around the proximal phalanx forming an expansion or a "hood" (Fig. 1–78). This hood goes around the phalanx and attaches to the transverse metacarpal ligament (Fig. 1–79).

The intrinsic muscles originate in the palmar aspect of the hand and pass to the dorsum of the extensor apparatus. They pass "palmar" to the joint fulcrum of the metacarpophalangeal joint and thus flex this joint (Fig. 1–80). They then pass "dorsal" to the fulcrum of the proximal and distal interphalangeal joints and extend these joints. As the proximal interphalangeal joint is brought into extension the retinacular ligament is placed under tension and extends the distal interphalangeal joint. This is the tenodesis action that remains controversial.[14] The two joints move in concert and always at the same angle.[14]

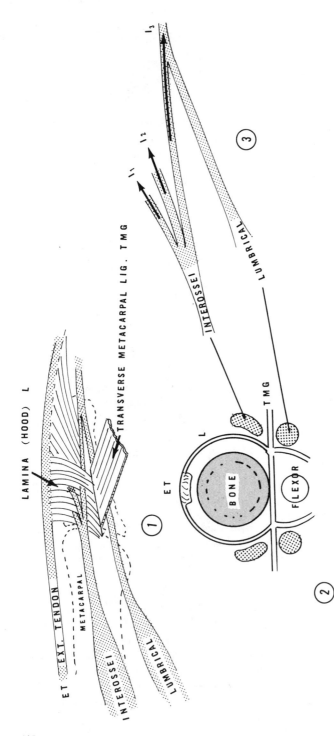

Figure 1-78. Extensor expansion detailed (the hood). (1) As the extensor tendon passes the end of the metacarpal, it expands into a flattened tissue resembling fascia and wraps around the proximal phalanx forming a hood. The interosseous muscle tendon divides into three slips—I_1 inserting into the bone which allows lateral finger motion (abduction-adduction); I_2 inserts into the lamina, thus stabilizing the extensor tendon; and I_3 proceeds to unite with the lumbrical tendon (which has passed under the transverse metacarpal ligament) to merge with the lateral bands of the extensor expansion. (2) Graphic cross section showing the two intrinsic muscles, the transverse ligament (TMG), the extensor tendon (ET), and the palmar longitudinal septum that encircles the flexor tendons. (3) Graphic view of the distribution of the interossei and lumbrical tendons as noted in (1).

Figure 1–79. Extensor of metacarpophalangeal joint. Action of the transverse lamina (hood) upon the phalanges. (A) The finger is in neutral position. The transverse lamina is relaxed permitting the digits to be moved laterally by the interossei. In this position the collateral ligaments are also relaxed (see Fig. 1–46). (B) The finger is shown in hyperextended position. The extensor tendon displaces the lamina proximally. As the proximal phalanx extends, the volar ligament is moved distally. The lamina becomes taut helping to extend the proximal phalanx. The oblique proximal fibers that attach from the extensor tendon and the lamina to the metacarpal neck periosteum are slackened. (C) In full flexion the extensor ten-

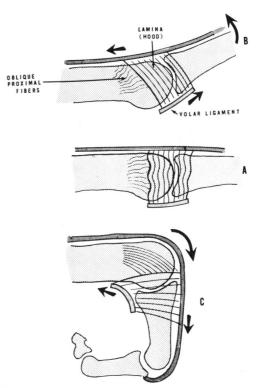

don moves distally causing the fibers of the lamina and the oblique proximal fibers to become taut. The flexor tendon moves the volar ligament proximally. This motion stabilizes the joint and fixes the extensor tendon. The oblique fibers limit the extent of motion of the extensor tendon.

It has been claimed that the oblique retinacular ligament extends the distal joint from 90° to 45° and the lateral bands from 45° to full extension (0°), but this proposition has been disproved[15] since, after section of the retinacular ligament, there was found to be no loss of extension from 7° to 90°. This finding led to the conclusion that "active extension of the distal phalanx was caused entirely by the lateral band, and the retinacular ligaments merely acted to maintain the central position of the extensor tendon." The hood was considered to be the most effective extensor of the proximal phalanx.

In forceful gripping, primarily a function of the extrinsic flexors, an unusual amount of electromyographic activity is noted in the extensors.[16] This extensor activity is considered to prevent palmar subluxation of the metacarpophalangeal joints during forceful gripping.

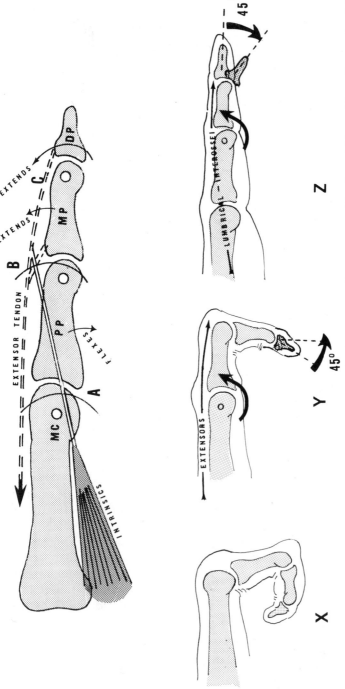

Figure 1–80. Action of the long extensors and intrinsics. (A) The intrinsics (interossei and lumbricals) lie on the palmar side of the metacarpophalangeal joint and thus flex this joint. (B) They pass to the dorsum of the fulcrum of the proximal interphalangeal joint and extend this joint. (C) The intrinsics attach to the extensors which in turn attach to the distal phalanx extending this joint (distal interphalangeal). The interossei and lumbricals cannot extend the interphalangeal joints (B) and (C) unless the metacarpophalangeal joint (A) is stabilized by the extensor tendon. (X) Depicts flexed finger. (Y) Flexing the proximal interphalangeal joint extends distal phalanx 45° by means of ligamentous action. (Z) Extending the proximal joint permits flexion of the interphalangeal joint 45°, indicating laxity of Landmeer's ligament.

60

The extensor tendons of the index and little fingers are joined on their medial sides at the metacarpophalangeal joints with isolated tendons: the extensor indicis to the index and the extensor digiti minimi to the fifth finger. The former enters the same fibrous tunnel as the common tendons, whereas the extensor digit quinti has its own sheath. As the extensor digitorum tendon to the fifth finger is often a frail slip, the extensor digit minimi is the main extensor of the little finger.

Intrinsic Muscles of the Thenar and Hypothenar Groups. The thenar muscles move the thumb and include the following (Fig. 1–81):

1. Abductor pollicis brevis. This muscle originates from the tubercle of the scaphoid ridge of the trapezium and the transverse carpal ligament. It inserts into the radial aspect of the base of the proximal phalanx of the thumb, and functions to abduct the thumb to the plane of the palm (Fig. 1–82).

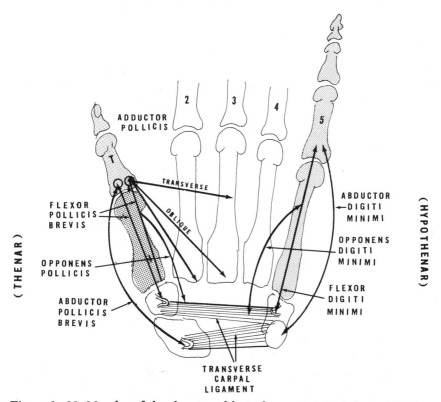

Figure 1–81. Muscles of the thenar and hypothenar regions (schematic). The muscles moving the thumb and little finger are shown. Only the intrinsic muscles are shown.

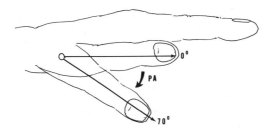

Figure 1-82. Palmar abduction. The range of passive or active palmar abduction from the plane of the palm, without any rotation of the thumb, should be 70°.

2. Flexor pollicis brevis. Originating from the ridge of the trapezium and the transverse carpal ligament, it inserts into the radial side of the base of the proximal phalanx. It also sends an insertion into the extensor expansion. There is a deep portion that originates from the base of the metacarpal that inserts into the ulnar sesamoid.
3. Opponens pollicis. Originating from the ridge of the trapezium and the transversecarpal ligament, it inserts along the entire margin of the first metacarpal. In its course it lies beneath the abductor pollicis brevis and the flexor pollicis brevis. This muscle flexes the proximal thumb joint (Fig. 1-83).
4. Abductor pollicis. Its "transverse" portion originates from the third metacarpal and inserts into the ulnar sesamoid of the thumb. Its "oblique" portion arises from the bases of the second and third metacarpals and the capitate bone to insert into the ulnar sesamoid. This muscle also abducts the thumb against the plane of the palm.

The hypothenar muscles move the little finger and include the following:

1. Abductor digiti minimi. Originating from the pisiform bone, it inserts into the ulnar aspect of the base of the proximal phalanx of the fifth finger. It abducts the little finger against the plane of the palm.
2. Flexor digiti minimi. Originating from the hook of the hamate and the transverse carpal ligament, it inserts into the ulnar side of the base of the proximal phalanx of the little finger. It flexes the proximal phalanx of the little finger.
3. Opponens digiti minimi. It originates from the hood of the hamate and the transverse carpal ligament. It inserts along the ulnar side of the fifth metacarpal. In its course it lies under the abductor digiti minimi and the flexor digiti minimi. This muscle opposes the little fingertip against the tip of the thumb (Fig. 1-84).

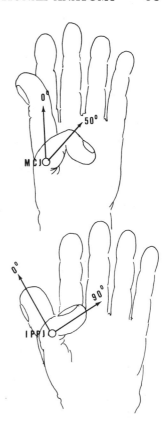

Figure 1–83. Measurement of thumb flexion. The upper figure depicts the range of flexion of the thumb at the metacarpal joint (0° to 50°). The lower figure depicts flexion at the thumb interphalangeal joints (IPPJ) which normally is 0° to 90°.

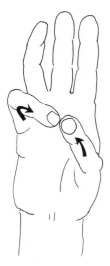

Figure 1–84. Opposition of the thumb and little finger. Palmar view of opposition with the thumb tip touching the tip of the little finger. The thenar and hypothenar muscles can be tested by resisting this motion. Once opposed these muscles can be tested.

4. Palmaris brevis. It originates from the transverse carpal ligament and inserts into the skin of the hand on the ulnar side.

The movements resulting from the thenar and hypothenar muscles are complex and require definition (see Fig. 1–40). The names of the individual muscles actually designate their function. Thus "pollicis" implies the thumb and "digiti minimi" the little (fifth) finger.

The thumb moves upon the saddle-shaped joint of the trapezium (see Fig. 1–42). Opposition of the thumb is a combination of all motions. It begins as extension proceeding to abduction, then becomes flexion into adduction. The reverse occurs in the return to neutral position.

There is a difference between firm opposition and soft opposition, with the former being primarily from action of the flexor pollicis brevis.

TECHNIQUES OF EXAMINATION

The manner of dividing the hand into zones varies with the clinician. The following is an acceptable classification, with numbered zones on the ulnar side and T-enumerated zones for the thumb (Fig. 1–85).

The soft tissues contained within precise zones require individual descriptions. Many of the tissues within these zones that must be recognized for a meaningful clinical examination are tendons.

Tendons can be readily palpated, as many are present directly under the skin. As a consequence of their attachment from a muscle group to a specific point upon a bone, their main function is to effect a precise motion. That precise motion not only contracts a specific muscle but makes the tendon taut and therefore palpable. Clinical examination demands that the precise muscle be identified, and the tendon be examined for integrity, by precise muscle contraction.

Precise examination of the muscles, their tendons, and their nerve supply is described and illustrated in Chapter 2.

The various ranges of motion of the numerous joints of the fingers are described below.

Flexion-Extension of the Metacarpophalangeal Joints

These joints can be tested individually or together. The examiner stabilizes the hand by firmly holding the hand across the palm (i.e., the metacarpal bones). The fingers at their proximal phalanges move in extension and flexion upon the metacarpal heads (the knuckles).

Figure 1-85. Anatomical zones of tendon injuries. Zone I is at the DIP joint level and Zone 8 (not shown) is at the distal forearm level. Muscular injuries occur proximal to Zone 8 and tendons at Zone 7 and 8 are beneath subcutaneous, reticulum and fascial levels.

The tendons at Zone 6 are very superficial and are relatively round or oval lacerations at zone 5 are at the MP joint level. Tendons at this level usually do not retract. Zones 4 and 3 are at the Interphalangeal joint level and rarely include complete lacerations of the dorsal apparatus. Lacerations at zones 2 and 1 are conceptually simple: thin and oriented upon the dorsal aspect of the middle phalanx. The thumb zones (TI-V) are discussed in the text.

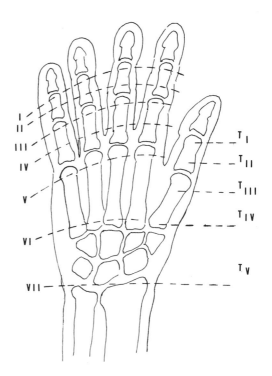

Flexion is normally 90°, with some hyperextension to 30°–45°. Abduction-adduction of the metacarpal-proximal phalangeal joint is possible to 20° in both directions, as the collateral ligaments are slack in the extended position. In the flexed position the collateral ligaments are taut by virtue of the ovoid nature of the metacarpal head.

Clinically the range of motion is determined by abducting and adducting the extended finger, then performing the same maneuver with the finger flexed to 90°. No significant motion is possible in the latter position (Fig. 1–86).

Phalangeal Joints. The proximal phalangeal joints flex normally to 100° and extend 0°. The distal interphalangeal joints flex 90° and extend to 20°. Due to their articular configurations there is no significant abduction or adduction of the these joints. There is normally 20° of abduction and adduction of the metacarpal phalangeal joints.

Thumb. The metacarpal phalangeal joint of the thumb flexes normally 50° with no (0°) extension. The interphalangeal joint flexes 90° and extends 20°. The thumb abducts 70°, with no (0°) adduction.

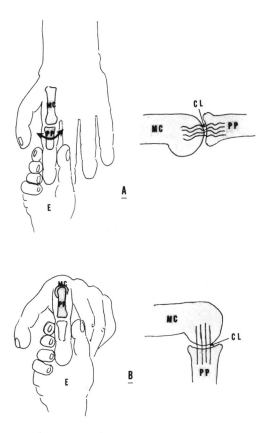

Figure 1–86. Examination of the metacarpal proximal-phalangeal joint. In the upper figure (A) the index finger is extended allowing passive motion of the metacarpal (MC) proximal-phalangeal (PP) joint (curved arrow). This motion is possible in that with the joint in extension the collateral ligaments (CL) are slack. With the finger flexed 90° (B) the collateral ligaments are taut by virtue of the head of the metacarpal being ovoid rather than round.

Flexibility of the Intrinsics. The intrinsics, which are finger extensors (see Fig. 1–80), can contract if not periodically elongated or if diseased. If limitations of the intrinsics exist and are responsible for limited joint range of motion that prevents full finger flexion, this must be ascertained and documented (Fig. 1–83). This test is termed the Bunnel-Littler Test (Fig. 1–87).

To perform this test the metacarpophalangeal joint is held at a few degrees of extension and the proximal phalanx is flexed. Normally the phalanx will flex, but if the intrinsics are "tight" the phalanx will not flex.

Differentiation of limitation due to joint capsular tightness from intrinsic tightness requires the test to be performed with a few degrees of flexion of the metacarpophalangeal joint so as to relax the intrinsics.

Examination of the wrist and fingers must always evaluate the passive and active range of motion of each joint in the hand. The examination must evaluate the capsular tissues of each joint, the precise mus-

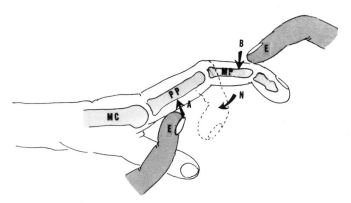

Figure 1-87. Bunnel-Littler test for intrinsic tightness. The examiner (E) slightly dorsiflexes the proximal phalanx (A) and the attempts to flex the phalanges (MP); (B). If there is tightness no flexion occurs. If the intrinsics are not tight the phalanges flex normally (N). MC is the metacarpal.

cle(s) involved, the adequacy of the tendons if present, and the nerve control. Merely doing an anatomical examination is meaningless unless the function is considered.

REFERENCES

1. Bowers WH, Tribuzi SM: Functional Anatomy. In: Stanley BG, Tribuzi M: Concepts in Hand Rehabilitation CPR. FA Davis, Philadelphia, 1992, pp 8-9.
2. John DA, Mennell J McM: Diagnosis and Physical Treatment. Musculoskeletal Pain. Little Brown, Boston, 1976, pp 8-9.
3. Mennell JM: Joint Pain. Boston Little Brown, 1964.
4. Cailliet R.: Mechanics of joints. In Licht S (ed): Arthritis and Physical Medicine, Vol 11. Waverly Press, Baltimore, 1969, pp 17-34.
5. Lampe EW: Surgical anatomy of the hand. Clin Symp CIBA 9:1957.
6. Thomas CL (ed): Taber's Cyclopedic Medical Dictionary, ed 16. FA Davis, Philadelphia, 1989, p 1833.
7. Lenman JAR: Clinical Neurophysiology. Blackwell, Edinburgh, 1975, p 95.
8. McMahon TA: Muscle, Reflexes and Locomotion. Princeton University Press, Princeton, N.J., 1984, p 172.
9. Long C: Intrinsic-extrinsic muscle control of the fingers. J Bone Joint Surg 50A:973, 1968.
10. Long C, Brown ME: Electromyographic kinesiology of the hand. Part III: lumbricalis and flexor digitorum profundus tote long finger. Arch Phys Med Rehabil 43:450, 1962.
11. Zancolli E: Structural and Dynamic Base of Hand Surgery. JB Lippincott, Philadelphia, 1968.

12. Landsmeer JMF: The anatomy of the dorsal aponeurosis of the human finger and its functional significance. Anat Rec 104:31, 1949.
13. Zancoli E: The lateral retinacular ligaments and the functional circuit of the fingers. In: Structural and Dynamic Bases of Hand Surgery. JB Lippincott, Philadelphia, 1968, pp 85–97.
14. Stack HG: Muscle function in the fingers. Bone Joint Surg 44B:899, 1962.
15. Harris R: Physical methods in the management of rheumatoid arthritis. Med Clin North Am 52:707, 1968.
16. Long C: Intrinsic-extrinsic muscle control of the fingers. J Bone Joint Surg 50A:973, 1968.

CHAPTER 2

Nerve Control of the Hand

Before initiating neuromuscular hand-finger activities, cortical activity is needed to place the hand where it is functionally needed. The planning steps that intervene between the decision and its initiation have long been the study of neurophysiologists.[1] The central nervous system is organized into densely interconnected population of neurons, many of which are hand related (Fig. 2-1).

The development of the hand is intimately related to the development of the neocortex; both of these serve to different humans from other primates. The intricate motor activities of the human hand in its numerous activities demand intricate cortical patterns that have evolved from basic patterns of mere grasp (Fig. 2-2).

Upper cortical patterns are directed through middle supraspinal centers into the final motor patterns of the cord (Fig. 2-3), and incorporate sensory feedback (Fig. 2-4).

It has been ascertained that sensory feedback is necessary for precise neuromusculoskeletal activities.[2] In animal experiments, the postcentral cortex devoted to the fingers (Fig. 2-5) has been found to show increased activity during learning tasks.[3] Furthermore, after the loss of peripheral innervation, a "remapping" of the cortical neurons has been documented.[4] This indicates that the previously held concept in which the brain is "hardwired" into unchangeable patterns is no longer tenable. The network of neuronal patterns is apparently continually remodeling itself and provides a basis for learning and retraining.

Discoveries have been based on clinical lesions in humans. For instance, misreaching and a lack of spatiomotor coordination has been noted as a result of a lesion of the parietal cortex, and deficits in learning or retrieval have been associated with lesions of the prefrontal and premotor cortex.

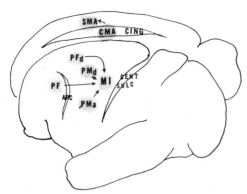

Figure 2–1. Arm related neuronal populations in the cerebral cortex (macaque monkey). The primary motor cortex (MI) located anterior to the central sulcus (Cent sulc) is 'fed' by dispersed neuronal populations as is the supplementary motor cortex (SMA) located in the region of the cingulate (CING) region. Some of these areas are PMd, PMa, and PFd in the post arcuate premotor cortex (arc) and PF in the prefrontal cortex area. CMA is a cingulate motor contex. The arrows indicate internucial linkage. Clinical manifestations from lesions of these areas indicate their specific shoulder-hand-finger motor functions. (Modified from Kalaska and Crammond.[1])

Painful lesions, as well as their sensory localization within the cortex, have been documented by magnetic resonance imaging (MRI) and positron emission tomography (PET) in humans.[5]

The present theory in which the brain functions as a simple passive receiver of information from the outside world, a theory which evolved from the simplistic legacy of Descartes (Fig. 2–6), is no longer tenable. Melzack postulates that pain patterns are present in a brain "substrate" of genetic origin, which is modified by experience.[6] The substrate, which he terms the "neuromatrix," is a network of neurons (loops) between the thalamus and the cortex. The cyclic processing and synthesis of impulses through this matrix form a "neurosignature." These neurosignatures evolve into awareness, which conveys the peripheral sensations in some instances into pain.

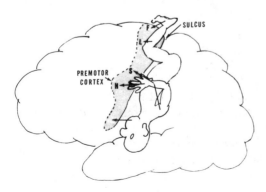

Figure 2–2. Premotor cortex (schematic).

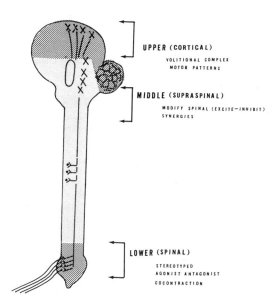

Figure 2–3. Central nervous system.

Sensorimotor systems for intricate activities have also been postulated and are currently well recognized. The spindle system that exists in all neuromuscular systems (Fig. 2–7) is predominant in the muscles responsible for hand-finger functions. All nonfusiformal muscles have intrafusal muscle spindles (Fig. 2–8) that monitor and coordinate motor activities. The Golgi organs of the tendons also are involved in neuromuscular coordination.

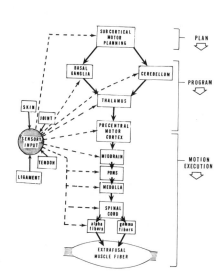

Figure 2–4. Spinal and supraspinal motor centers. (Adapted from Schmidt RF: Fundamentals of Neurophysiology. Springer-Verlag, New York, 1978.)

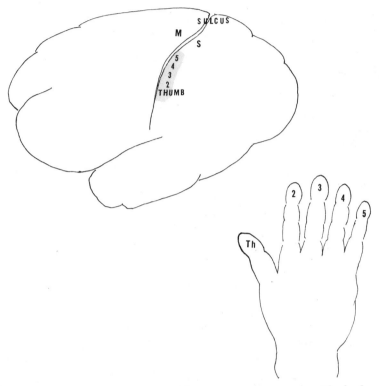

Figure 2–5. Finger representation in the somatosensory cortex. The body parts are represented in the somatosensory cortex in which the fingers and lips have larger representation. The five fingers numbered in the somatosensory cortex are shown posterior to the sulcus. Training of digital activities in monkeys have shown an enlargement of the areas. M depicts the motor aspect of the cortex and S the sensory.

Each muscle spindle is enclosed within a fascia that limits elongation (Fig. 2–9) and is thus involved in neuromuscular function.

BRACHIAL PLEXUS

From the cord, the nerve roots emerge to their muscular destiny (Fig. 2–10). In their extraspinal course they form the brachial plexus (Fig. 2–11). Any loss of hand function must therefore consider the neural pathways going to a specific muscle involved in a precise function from the cortex, the cord, the plexus, and the individual nerve. Evaluation of hand function addresses the peripheral mechanisms but must also consider more proximal neural circuits.

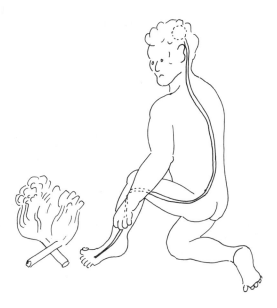

Figure 2–6. Kneeling man perceiving pain (Descartes). The Descartes kneeling figure (1596–1650) depicts a burning sensation irritating the filaments of a nerve in the foot ascending to the brain via the filaments of that nerve. (Rene Descartes' illustration from "De l'Homme" was modified by the author.)

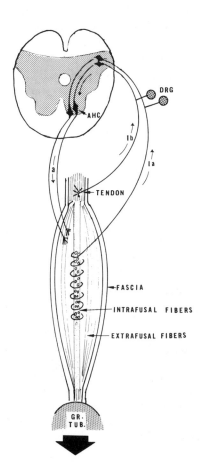

DRG

AHC

Ib

Ia

a

TENDON

FASCIA

INTRAFUSAL FIBERS

EXTRAFUSAL FIBERS

GR. TUB.

Figure 2–7. Spindle system function. The spindle system (intrafusal fibers) is parallel with the extrafusal fibers. When stretched, they signal the cord by way of Ia (from the spindle) and Ib (from the Golgi tendon organs) through the dorsal root ganglia (DRG). An interneural connection to the anterior horn cells (AHC) causes appropriate contraction of the extrafusal fibers. The fascia elongates according to its physiologic limits. In this illustration the muscle is the supraspinatus attached to the greater tuberosity (Gr. Tub.) of the humerus.

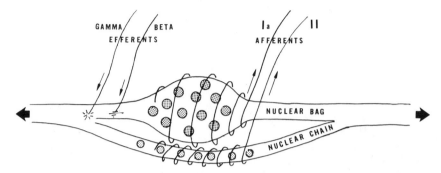

Figure 2 – 8. Intrafusal muscle spindle. The intrafusal spindle system has motor fibers through the gamma and beta efferents that control the length of the spindle. The sensory feedback from the spindle is transmitted by way of the Ia and II afferent fibers.

The peripheral nerve (Fig. 2 – 12) is often involved in loss of hand-finger function, and external forces to the peripheral nerve(s) are often responsible for loss of this function.

Five degrees of nerve damage have been documented by Sunderland (Fig. 2 – 13) and these remain the basis for clinical grading.[7]

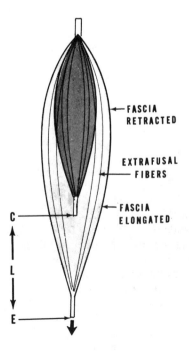

Figure 2–9. Fascial limits to muscular elongation. Any muscle bundle will elongate to the extent that its fascial sheath will permit. The extrafusal fibers elongate fully, but the fascia must passively be elongated. It is fascial contracture that restricts muscular elongation and joint range of motion.

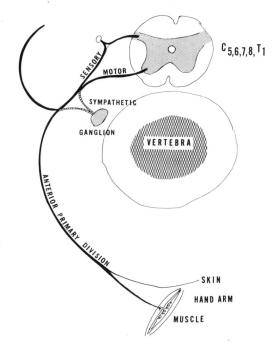

$C_{5,6,7,8}, T_1$

SENSORY

MOTOR

SYMPATHETIC

GANGLION

VERTEBRA

ANTERIOR PRIMARY DIVISION

SKIN

HAND ARM

MUSCLE

Figure 2-10. Nerve root. The nerve root—its sensory, motor, and sympathetic components—is shown as to its anterior primary division. The posterior primary division, with its branches to the skin, neck posterior muscles, and zyoapophyseal joints, is not depicted.

First degree injury constitutes loss of conductivity of the axon without loss of continuity in the axon structure. A loss of motor function and tone with reduction of proprioception usually results, but touch and pain sensation remain.

Second degree injuries sever the axon with resultant wallerian degeneration. The endoneural tubes remain intact and permit axons to regenerate within their own tubules. Within 20 hours there is complete sensorimotor and sympathetic loss (Fig. 2-14), and there is no reaction to electrical stimulation. Motor atrophy ensues and chromatolysis occurs, with degeneration of the anterior horn cell or the posterior root of the sensory nerve. As the nerve root is more involved than is the anterior horn cell, there is greater sensory then motor loss, and recovery of sensation is slower than motor recovery. Regardless of surgical intervention (suture) recovery is the norm.

Third degree injury disorganizes the internal structure of the funiculus and thus interrupts both the axon and the tubule. The epineurium and perineurium remain intact. The usual hemorrhage occurring within the funiculus causes "fibrosis," which complicates the ultimate recovery. The residual loss depends on the site of injury; the more distal the injury the less the loss in function.

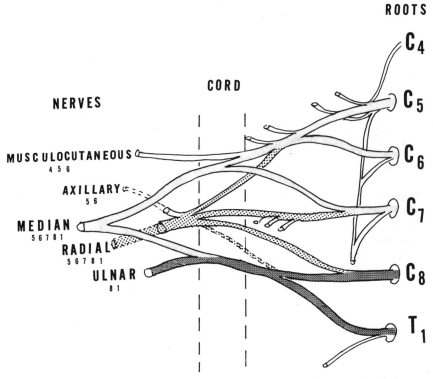

Figure 2-11. Brachial plexus (schematic). The brachial plexus is divided into roots, cords, and the five major nerves (with their root components).

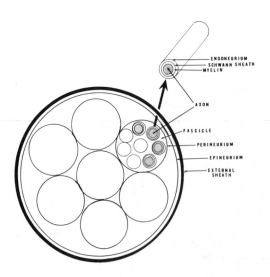

Figure 2-12. Cross section of a peripheral nerve. A nerve is composed of numerous axones grouped within a fascicle. Each axone is surrounded by myelin enclosed within a sheath of Schwann. These sheaths are coated with endoneurium composed of longitudinal collagen sheaths. A perineurium sheath contains these fascicles in bundles. Numerous fascicles are bound by epineureum, which are totally covered by an external sheath.

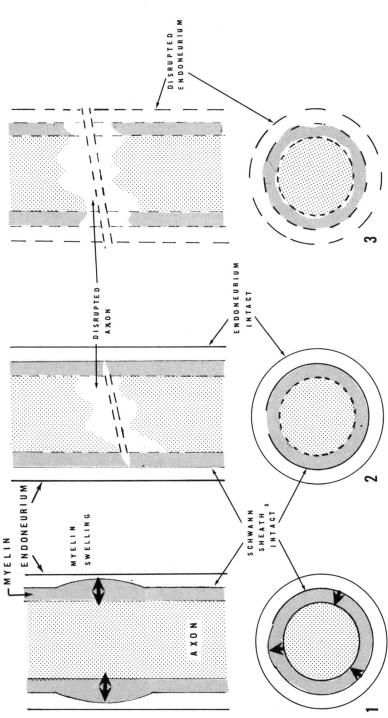

Figure 2–13. Degrees of nerve injury. (1) A loss of conductivity "without" break in continuity. The myelin swells within an intact Schwann sheath that compresses the axon (arrows). (2) The axon is severed but the endoneural sheath (tubule) remains intact as may the Schwann sheath. The axon regenerates within its own tubule. (3) The entire fascicle, the axon, Schwann sheath and endoneurium, is disrupted. Regeneration is usually prevented by fibrosis occurring at the severed ends.

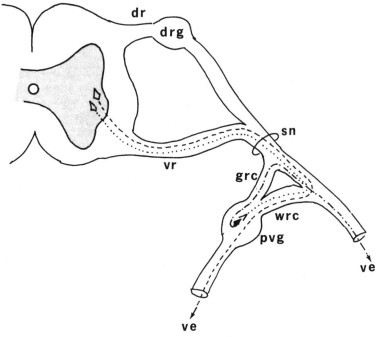

Figure 2–14. Autonomic fibers in a spinal nerve. The lateral horn cells from which emerge the autonomic nerves are located in the gray matter of the cord. The dorsal root ganglia (DRG) is the site of emergence of the somatic nerves (DR). The afferent autonomic nerves emerge via the ventral root on to the spinal nerve (SN), which then proceeds to the paravertebral ganglia (PVG). The preganglionic fibers enter the ganglia through the white ramus communicans (WRC) where some proceed without synapse and others synapse to reenter the spinal nerve through the gray ramus communications (GRC). These proceed down the primary division of the nerve root. (VE = visceral efferent nerves.)

Fourth and fifth degree injuries disrupt "all" funicular sheaths and cause a total loss of motor, sensory, and sympathetic function. The nerve is "divided," with a resultant neuroma forming at the end. Even under optimal conditions limited recovery of function is the norm.

The degrees of disruption have been termed as

1. *Neuropraxia*—physiological interruption (discrete demyelination) with intact nerve and no wallerian degeneration.[8,9]
2. *Axonotmesis*—axon disruption with degeneration but intact sheaths.[8] Degeneration of the axons and myelin sheaths distal to the lesion begins within 48 hours.
3. *Neurotmesis*—disruption of both axon and sheath.

After axonometric nerve injury the cell bodies (sensory nerves) located in the dorsal root ganglion or in the anterior horn of the spinal cord (motor) undergo a process called chromatolysis.[10] In this process the cell body swells, there is a proliferation of glial cells and a loss of Nissl bodies. All these changes occur within 7 days of the injury.

During degeneration, a reaction occurs within the anterior horn cell within 2 to 3 weeks from a substance termed "axoplasm" that stimulates distal growth. The proximal stump produces a number of terminal and collateral processes, which grow at a rate of 1 mm per day toward the distal nerve segment.[10] Some of these processes may be misdirected to produce neuromas. Growth of these terminal processes is influenced by the presence of nerve growth factor (NGF).[11]

Loss of motor and sensory function are apparent, but the occurrence of sympathetic pain and dysfunction after nerve injury have become more widely recognized[12] (Fig. 2–15). Sympathetic maintained

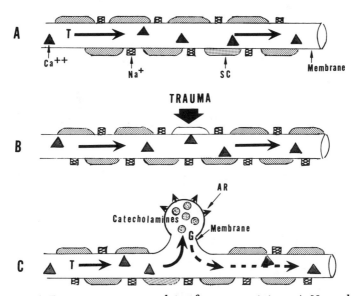

Figure 2–15. Ectopic generator evolving from nerve injury. A, Normal nerve, which is a transmitter (T) of impulses within the membrane (M). The Schwann cells (SC) of the membrane form the myelin sheath. The electrolytes sodium (Na^+) and Calcium (Ca^{++}) generate the impulse. B, Trauma damages the Schwann cells of the membrane. C, At the site of trauma there is a release of catecholamines, and the membrane forms a saccule containing these catecholamines, which become generators (G) of abnormal impulses (*broken line*). Adrenergic receptors (AR) form on the membrane surface of the saccule explaining the hypersensitivity of the nerve at that site. (Modified from Devor M: Nerve pathophysiology and mechanisms of pain in causalgia. J Autonom Nerv Sys 7:371–384, 1983.)

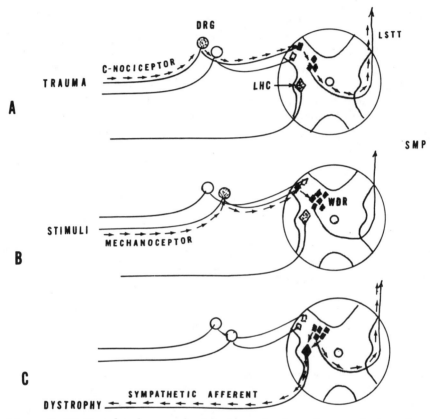

Figure 2–16. Postulated neurophysiologic mechanism of sympathetic maintained pain (SMP). The transmission via C-nociceptor fibers (A) of impulses from the peripheral tissues that have been traumatized and created peripheral nociceptor chemicals (see details in text). These impulses pass through the dorsal root ganglion (DRG) to activate the gray matter of the cord in the Rexed layers. When sensitized, they are termed *wide dynamic range (WDR) neurons.* The WDR, becoming very irritated, receives impulses from the periphery via the A-mechanoreceptor fibers (*B*), which normally transmit sensations of touch, vibration, temperature, and so on. When the periphery is stimulated (skin touch, pressure, or joint movement), these impulses enhance and maintain the irritability of the WDR. The impulses from the WDR continue cephalad through the lateral spinothalamic tracts (LSTTs) to the thalamic centers with resultant continued pain. The WDR impulses irritate the lateral horn cells (LHC), which generate sympathetic impulses that innervate the peripheral tissues, resulting in the symptoms and findings of dystrophy (*C*).

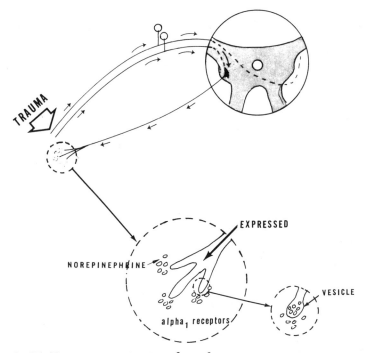

Figure 2–17. Nociceptor activation of α_1-adrenoreceptors. Trauma causes the sympathetic nerves going to the area to express norepinephrine that is contained within the vesicles. The liberated norepinephrine reacts with the α_1-receptors to create causalgic symptoms. Terminal vesicle can be considered a neuroma.

pain can result (Fig. 2–16) from axonometric nerve injury, or from nerve interruption due to a neuroma (Fig. 2–17).

CLINICAL EVALUATION
OF HAND FUNCTION

An adequate evaluation of hand function by means of a history and physical examination necessitates a thorough neurological examination of the extremity. Locating the site of disruption or nerve impairment must proceed by following the nerve pathway from the cerebral cortex to the cord, the brachial plexus, and ultimately the peripheral nerve. Examination is primarily manual, but ultimately diagnosis may be confirmed by more precise testing procedures.

Testing Procedures

The sensory tests can be neurophysiologically classified into four types: innervation density, threshold tests, stress tests, and sensory nerve conduction studies.

The motor tests involve manual resistance testing of individual muscle groups that have a specific nerve supply.

Innervation Density Test. This is a test for determining the ability to discriminate between two identical stimuli placed close together on the skin. Essentially it relates skin sensation with high-level cortical determination.[13] The more richly innervated the area being tested, the sharper is the contrast between the stimuli, and the more easily the brain can discriminate. A high level of cortical integrity is needed if this is to be a valid test of peripheral impairment.

Static two-point discrimination testing can be performed with an adjustable caliper (Fig. 2–18) or a similar device. Calipers can be adjusted to determine the precise width of the two contact points. Usually, an effective means of testing is to begin with a 2-mm separation of the contact points, applied parallel to the longitudinal axis on the palmar surface of the finger-tip. A straightened paper clip can be used. The values used are age dependent.[14]

Threshold Tests

Light-Touch Testing. Sensation of light touch can be tested with the use of a cotton swab, or more precisely by the use of a monofilament of

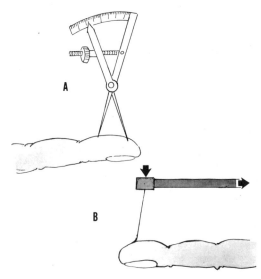

Figure 2–18. Light touch testing; caliper two-point test and Semmes-Weinstein monofilament discrimination test. *(A)* depicts the caliper that can be accurately used to measure two-point discrimination. *(B)* is the varied monofilaments that test for pressure of light touch discrimination.

varying thickness and inflexibility. A structured test set is the Semmes-Weinstein monofilament discrimination test.[15] Not only is light touch determined but the number of milligrams of force of the filament can be documented. This is a highly sophisticated test and is most valuable in determining recovery of a repaired severed nerve.

Vibration Testing. Sensation of vibration can be tested by direct application of a tuning fork or use of a Bio-Thesiometer, which records the quantitative voltage applied versus perceived vibratory stimulus.

Stress Tests. These tests are tests that provoke symptoms as a result of nerve compression. The tests are performed before and after significant pressure has been applied to the nerve being tested. Numerous stress tests will be discussed subsequently.

The Tinel sign[16] can be considered to be a stress test in that abrupt compression (digital tapping) of a nerve can elicit tingling in the skin along the course of the nerve.

Sensory Nerve Conduction Studies. These are electrophysiological instrument tests that assess conduction of sensory action potentials along a nerve trunk. The details and techniques are well documented in the medical literature.[17]

As the brachial plexus (Fig. 2–9) ultimately divides into five major nerves these will be individually discussed and their diagnostic procedures elicited. Sensory testing of dermatomes indicates the competence of the involved nerve, but motor (myotome) testing is more accurate in isolating the precise nerve involved or impaired. In clinical functional evaluation, it behooves the examiner to understand the precise muscle(s) specifically innervated by a single nerve and its roots.

THE MEDIAN NERVE

The median nerve originates from roots C_6, C_7, C_8, and T_1. It descends down the inner aspect of the upper arm and enters the forearm by passing between the ulnar and humeral heads of the pronator teres, where it gives off the anterior interrosseous branch (Fig. 2–19).

The muscles innervated by the median nerve emanating from roots C_6, C_7, C_8, and T_1 are listed in Fig. 2–20. Each muscle innervated by the median nerve can be manually tested to determine the integrity of the nerve.

The muscles innervated by the median nerve are listed and illustrated below:

1. Pronator teres (C_6, C_7), which pronates the forearm (Fig. 2–21).
2. Flexor carpi radialis (C_6, C_7, C_8), which flexes the wrist in a radial direction (Fig. 2–22).

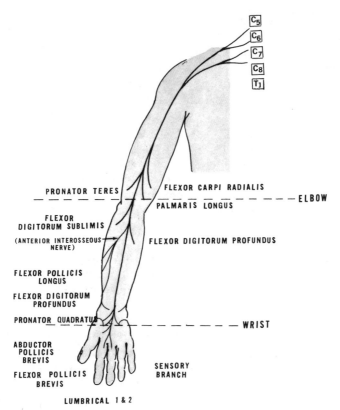

Figure 2-19. Median nerve.

ROOTS			
C6	C7	C8	T1
FL. CARPI RADIALIS			
PRONATOR TERES			
	ABD. POLL. LONGUS		
	PALMARIS LONGUS		
	PRONATOR QUADRATUS		
	FL. DIGITORUM SUBLIMIS		
	FL. DIGITORUM PROFUNDUS		
	FL. POLLICIS LONGUS		
		OPPONENS POLL	
		ABD. POLL. BREV.	
		FL. POLLICIS BREVIS	

Figure 2-20. Cervical root component of the median nerve.

MEDIAN NERVE C_6
                C_7

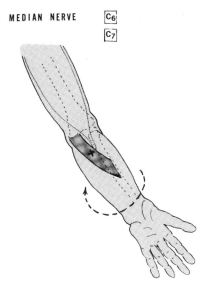

Figure 2–21. Pronator teres. The pronator teres is supplied by the median nerve of cervical roots C_6 and C_7. Its function is to pronate the forearm. "X" denotes its motor point or EMG diagnostic site. The muscle originates from the medial epicondyle of the humerus and the coronoid process of the ulna. It inserts into the midshaft of the radius.

MEDIAN NERVE

C_6

C_7

C_8

MEDIAL
EPICONDYLE

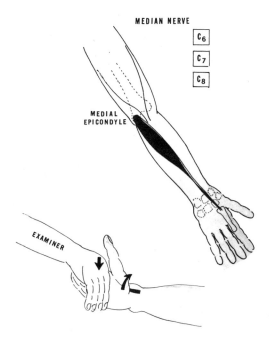

EXAMINER

Figure 2–22. Flexor carpi radialis. The flexor carpi radialis flexes the wrist in a radial direction. The tendon is palpable at wrist (see Fig. 1–23). Muscle originates from medial epicondyle of the humerus. The flexor carpi radialis is innervated by median nerve cervical roots C_6, C_7, and C_8. It inserts upon the volar surface of the base of the second metacarpal, and is best examined with the forearm supinated.

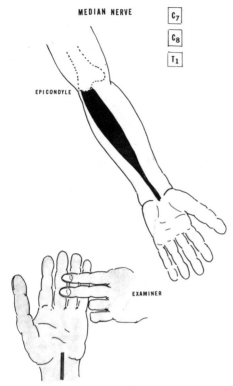

MEDIAN NERVE

C_7

C_8

T_1

EPICONDYLE

EXAMINER

Figure 2-23. Palmaris longus. This muscle is supplied by the median nerve of cervical roots C_7, C_8 and T_1. It flexes the wrist, originates from the medial epicondyle of the humerus, and inserts into the palmar aponeurosis. "X" indicates the myoneural junction. In performing an EMG, if the needle is inserted too deeply, it may reach into the flexor digitorum sublimis, if too medial, into the flexor carpi ulnaris; and too radial, into the flexor carpi radialis.

3. Palmaris longus (C_7, C_8, T_1), which flexes the wrist (Fig. 2-23).
4. Flexor digitorum sublimis (C_7, C_8, T_1), which flexes the proximal interphalangeal joints (Fig. 2-24).

The anterior interrosseous branch of the median nerve supplies the following muscles:

1. Flexor pollicis longus (C_8, T_1), which flexes the distal digit of the thumb (Fig. 2-25).
2. Flexor digitorum profundus (C_8, T_1), which flexes the distal phalanx of the index (second) and middle (third) phalanx of the digit (Fig. 2-26).
3. Pronator quadratus (C_7, C_8, T_1) which pronates the forearm (Fig. 2-27).

As the median nerve descends the arm into the hand it passes, at the wrist, under the transverse carpal ligament through the carpal tunnel.

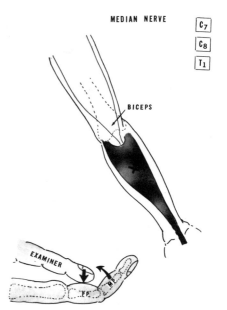

Figure 2–24. Flexor digitorum sublimis. This muscle flexes the proximal
interphalangeal joint. It is tested by
maintaining the proximal phalanx neutral. It originates from the medial epicondyle and coronoid process of the
ulna, and inserts upon the volar surface of the base of the second phalanx
(see Fig. 1–59).

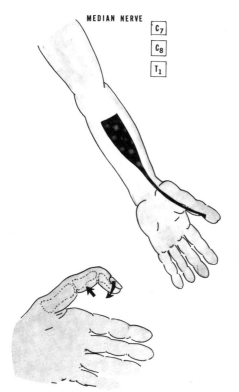

Figure 2–25. Flexor pollicis longus. This muscle flexes the distal
phalanx of the thumb. The flexor
tendon is not palpable. The muscle
originates from the volar surface of
the radius and inserts to the volar
surface of the base of the distal phalanx of the thumb. It is innervated
by the median nerve and roots C_7,
C_8, and T_1.

MEDIAN NERVE C_8 T_1

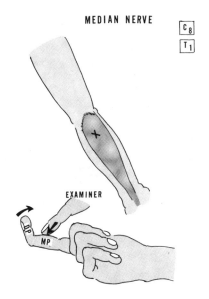

EXAMINER

Figure 2-26. Flexor digitorum profundus. Examiner restricts the middle phalanx flexion, and the flexor digitorum profundus flexes the distal phalanx.

There it splits into two branches, the lateral and medial branches, with variations to be discussed in a subsequent portion of this chapter.

The lateral branch is essentially motor and supplies the following muscles:

1. Abductor pollicis brevis (C_8, T_1), which elevates the thumb at a right angle to the plane of the palm (Fig. 2-28).

MEDIAN NERVE C_7 C_8 T_1

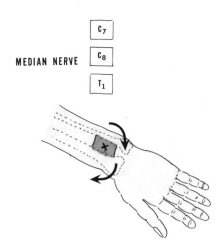

Figure 2-27. Pronator quadratus. The pronator quadratus is innervated by the median nerve (anterior interosseous nerve) roots C_7, C_8, and T_1. It originates from the lower quarter of the volar surface of the ulna and inserts into the lower quarter of the lateral volar surface of the radius; it also pronates the forearm.

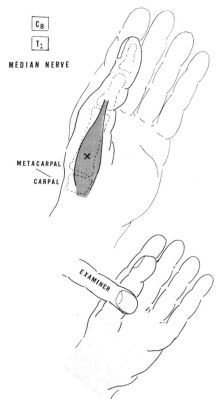

Figure 2–28. Abductor pollicis brevis. This muscle abducts the thumb in the palmar plane (see Fig. 1–40). It originates from the tubercle of the scaphoid and trapezium (see Fig. 1–81). It inserts upon the lateral base of the proximal phalanx of the thumb. This nerve is frequently used for nerve conduction tests (EMG) for carpal tunnel syndrome.

2. Flexor pollicis brevis (C_8, T_1), which flexes the metacarpophalangeal joint of the thumb (Fig. 2–29).
3. Opponens pollicis (C_8, T_1), which opposes the tip of the thumb to the tip of the little or first finger (Fig. 2–30).
4. First and second lumbricals.

Sensory Innervation of the Median Nerve

The dermatomal innervation of the hand from the median nerve is depicted in Fig. 2–31. Testing modalities have already been discussed.

Clinically, the degree of impairment from median nerve lesions depends upon the level of injury. The most common site is the wrist, where the nerve passes through the carpal tunnel. The mechanism of injury varies from a Colles' fracture, to tenosynovitis of the flexor tendons, rheumatoid arthritis, myxodema, or repetitive traumata.

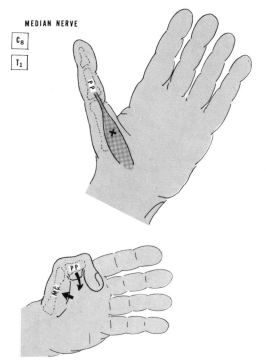

Figure 2–29. Flexor pollicis brevis. The flexor pollicis brevis flexes the proximal phalanx of the thumb. It is examined by restricting flexion of the metacarpal and is innervated by median nerve cervical roots C_8 and T_1. It originates from the ridge of the trapezium and transverse carpal ligament (see Fig. 1–81) and inserts on the radial side of the base of the proximal phalanx.

The history and physical examination may indicate paresthesia, hypalgesia, or hyperesthesia over the dermatomal distribution of the nerve. The motor loss varies from that of weakness of the involved muscles to clinical atrophy of the thenar eminence (Fig. 2–32).

A complete lesion of the median nerve at the wrist results in the following:

1. Inability to oppose the thumb.
2. Inability to abduct the thumb.
3. Atrophy of the thenar eminence.
4. Numbness of the dermatome region.

It must be recognized that as the patient can make a fist, specific motor testing is mandatory if the lesion is to be discovered.

Interruption of the median nerve "above" the elbow results in the partial inability to make a fist, as weakness results from involvement of the flexor digitorum sublimis; however, the other remaining flexors function. Pronation of the forearm is impaired and the wrist flexes in an ulnar direction. The distal phalanges do not flex, and remain extended,

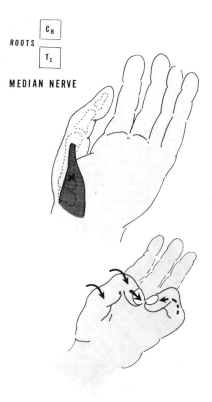

ROOTS $\boxed{C_8}$

$\boxed{T_1}$

MEDIAN NERVE

Figure 2-30. Opponens pollicis. The opponens pollicis originates from the tubercle of the trapezium. It inserts into the lateral half of the palmar aspect of the first metacarpal and is supplied by median nerve roots C_8, T_1. It opposes the thumb tip to little finger by rotating the first metacarpal (see Figs. 1-42 and 2-11).

with finger flexion occurring only at the middle phalangeal joint. It is therefore apparent that a careful muscle examination is needed to confirm the level of nerve involvement, as well as to specify "the" nerve involved.

A cord lesion involving specific root involvement (C_6, C_7, C_8, T_1) would cause weakness and nonspecific sensory involvement, as most finger motions have multiple root innervations. The root involvement most likely to simulate a median nerve lesion is C_8 (see Fig. 2-20).

In a cord lesion at the C_6 level, the shoulder is elevated and the arm abducted, due to paresis of the pectoral muscle (C_6–C_8), the latissimus dorsi (C_6–C_8), and the subscapularis (C_5–C_7). The elbow is flexed due to paresis of the triceps (C_6–C_8). All the muscles below C_6 are paralyzed, along with extensor carpi radialis longus; the triceps remains functional as there remains some innervation from C_6. Cord lesions at this level result in sensory loss of the entire hand, the fingers, and much of the forearm, as numerous dermatomes are involved.

A cord lesion at C_7 evoke the same arm posture as the C_6 lesion, but

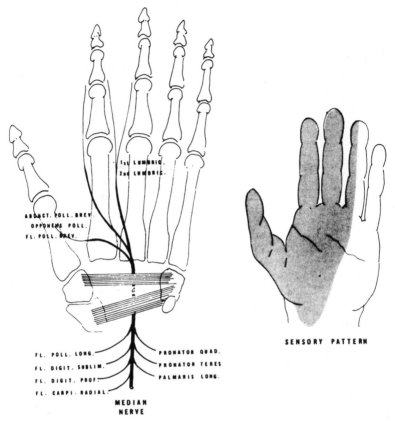

Figure 2–31. Median nerve. The motor branches of the median nerve are shown in the left figure; the right figure shows its sensory pattern.

the effects are less pronounced. In the hand, the extensor carpi radial longus remains functional, but the hand deviates in a radial direction. There is strength reduction in the pronator teres, flexor carpi radalis, flexor digitorum sublimis and profundus, and the flexor pollicis longus. The deep biceps and radial tendon reflexes remain active, but the finger flexor reflexes become hyperactive as supraspinal control is lost. With a C_7 lesion, sensory loss occurs at the inner aspect of the forearm and the ulnar side of the hand, with sparing of the median sensory pattern.

A C_8 cord lesion does not invoke a significant upper extremity posture, as the shoulder musculature remains balanced between internal and external rotators, abductors and adductors, and the elbow remains neutral, with a balance of the triceps and biceps. In the hand, the extensor pollicis brevis, interossei, opponens, and abductor pollicis

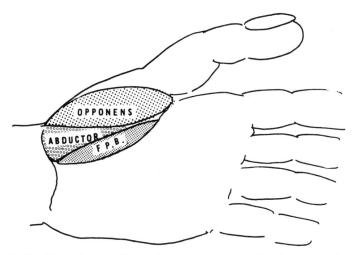

Figure 2–32. Musculature of the thenar eminence. The three muscles of the thenar eminence, innervated by the median nerve, are positioned as shown. This anatomic arrangement facilitates the insertion of EMG needles during diagnostic examination.

brevis are impaired. Because impairment of the interossei and lumbricals allows uncontrolled antagonistic action of the extensor digitorum communis and flexor digitorum sublimis and profundus, the hand assumes a "claw" position.

In the examination of the upper extremity of a patient with a T_1 cord lesion, only the hand is diagnostic. The flexor digitorum profundus and sublimis, flexor pollicis longus and brevis, extensor pollicis longus and brevis, abductor pollicis longus and opponens all function, with paresis only of the adductor pollicis interrosei and lumbricals. Ulnar sensation is apparent only in the forearm and the distal aspect of the upper arm, and is absent in the hand.

Proper, careful examination of the upper extremity, wrist, hand, and fingers, including motor function and sensory mapping, can precisely depict the exact site and specific nerve involvement of a lesion. A thorough knowledge of the functional anatomy of the hand is obviously mandatory, which is why this text places so much emphasis on functional anatomy.

ULNAR NERVE

The ulnar nerve is derived from two cervical nerve roots, C_8 and T_1 (Fig. 2–33), and is a continuation of the brachial plexus. It passes down

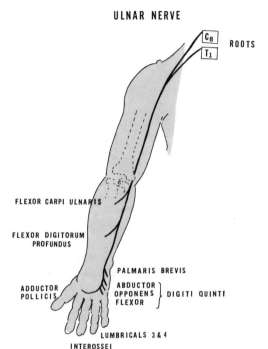

Figure 2-33. Ulnar nerve comprising roots C_8 and T_1.

the inner aspect of the upper arm in the proximity of the brachial artery lying between the biceps and triceps muscles. At the elbow it passes through a groove behind the medial epicondyle of the humerus.

In its passage along the ulnar aspect of the forearm the ulnar nerve supplies the following muscles:

1. Flexor carpi ulnaris (C_8, T_1), which flexes the wrist in an ulnar direction. It also flexes the wrist when it abducts the little finger (Fig. 2-34).
2. Flexor digitorum profundus (C_8, T_1), which flexes the distal digit of the little finger and usually the flexor of the distal digit of the ring finger. The latter is also often innervated by the median nerve (Fig. 2-35).

In the upper portion of the forearm, the ulnar nerve passes between the humeral and ulnar heads of the flexor carpi ulnaris muscle. It becomes superficial as it approaches the wrist, where it lies near the ulnar artery (see Fig. 1-23). Near the pisiform bone (see Fig. 1-8), the ulnar nerve gives off a palmar branch that innervates the skin of the ulnar aspect of the hand (Fig. 2-36), and a dorsal branch that innervates the ulnar aspect of the hand (Fig. 2-37).

ULNAR NERVE $\boxed{C_8}$
               $\boxed{T_1}$

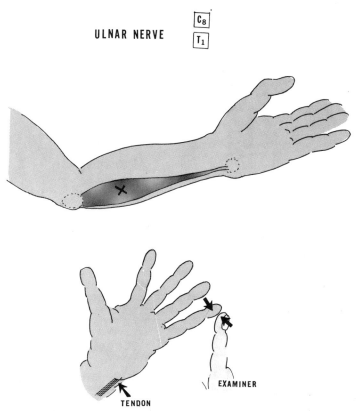

Figure 2–34. Flexor carpi ulnaris. It originates from the medial epicondyle of the humerus, medial of olecranon, and dorsal border of the ulna. It inserts into the pisiform (see Fig. 1–21) and flexes the wrist in an ulnar direction. It is innervated by ulnar nerve roots C_8, T_1. The examiner resists abduction and flexion of the fifth finger, which tenses the flexor carpi ulnaris at the pisiform (see Fig. 1–23).

As it rounds the hamate bone beneath the flexor digiti minimi muscle, the ulnar nerve divides into its terminal branches, which supply the following muscles:

1. Abductor digiti minimi (brevis), which abducts the little finger in the plane of the palm (see Fig. 1–40).
2. Opponens digit minimi, which opposes the little finger toward the thumb.
3. Adductor pollicis, which adducts the thumb in the plane of the palm.
4. Palmar interossei, which adduct the fingers toward the midline (see Fig. 1–67).

ULNAR NERVE $\boxed{C_8}$ $\boxed{T_1}$

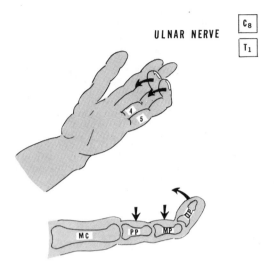

Figure 2–35. Flexor digitorum profundus. It flexes the distal phalanx and is tested by fixing the middle and proximal phalanx. It is supplied by ulnar nerve roots C_8, T_1. Muscle originates from the midulnar bone and interosseous membrane (see Fig. 1–56). It inserts into the base of the distal phalanx (see Fig. 1–59).

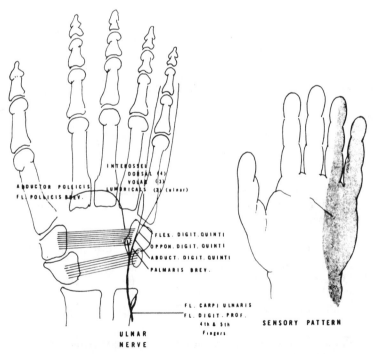

Figure 2–36. Ulnar nerve—motor and sensory distribution.

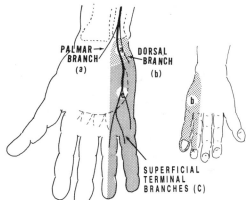

ULNAR NERVE
(SENSORY)

PALMAR (VIEWS) DORSAL

Figure 2-37. Ulnar nerve—sensory pattern.

The interossei can be tested by resisting the extended fingers in an opposing or approaching direction to/from the middle finger (see Fig. 1-70).

A severed ulnar nerve at the elbow causes the following clinical picture:

1. Flexion deformity of the fourth and fifth fingers (from paralysis of the lumbrical muscles).
2. Atrophy of the hypothenar eminence.
3. Atrophy of the interossei.
4. Atrophy of the web between the thumb and index finger (from paralysis of the first dorsal interosseus and adductor pollicis muscle).
5. Weakness of wrist flexion in an ulnar direction.
6. Weakness of flexion of the distal digit of the little finger.

Interruption of the ulnar nerve at the wrist causes weakness of abduction and adduction of the fingers and loss of adduction "sweep" of the thumb. This sweep is evident in that, normally, as the thumb adducts across the metacarpal heads it maintains contact with the skin of the palm.

Ulnar paralysis also results in the inability to grasp a piece of paper between the thumb and the radial side of the palm. This is termed a "positive Froment sign." Abduction of the index finger in the palmar plane is also lost.

When all the small muscles of the hand receive their innervation from the ulnar nerve this becomes an "all ulnar" hand and confuses the examiner.

Root Lesions: $C_8 - T_1$

Since all muscles innervated by C_8 also receive innervation from T_1 (Fig. 2–38), it is not possible to specify the location of a lesion to either root by examination of the hand muscles. A lesion specific to either will result in weakness but not paralysis.

Dermatomal evaluation of cervical lesions of C_8 or T_1 varies as noted in Fig. 2–39. A T_1 lesion involves the dermatome on the ulnar side of the forearm from the wrist to the elbow, whereas a C_8 lesion involves the ulnar aspect of the hand in both dorsal and palmar areas.

A cord lesion of C_8 and/or T_1 causes no abnormal posture of the upper extremity at the shoulder or elbow; the wrist is normal in regard to ulnar or radial deviation, and the finger flexor and thumb activities do

ROOTS			
C_6	C_7	C_8	T_1
		OPPONENS POLLICIS	
		ABDUCTOR POLLICIS BREVIS	
		FLEX. POLLICIS BREVIS	
		PALMAR BREVIS	
		ADDUCTOR POLLIC.	
		FLEX. DIGIT. MIN.	
		ABD. DIGIT. MIN.	
		OPPON. DIG. MIN.	
		INTEROSSEI	
		LUMBRICALS	

Figure 2–38. Ulnar nerve—cervical root component.

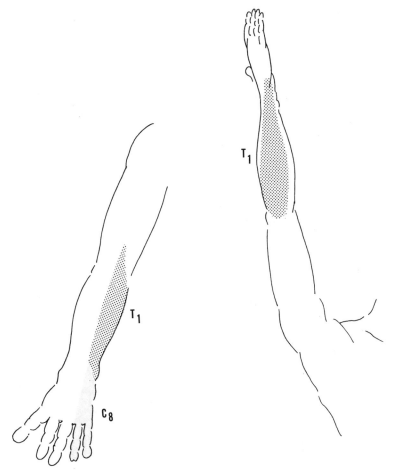

Figure 2–39. Sensory mapping of root lesions C_8 and T_1. The area of hypothesthesia clinically noted in root lesions of the eighth cervical and first thoracic is shown.

not change. The interossei and opponens, however, become reduced in strength, and because the abductor pollicis minimi becomes totally paralyzed the hand assumes a "clawed" appearance (from unopposed activity of the extensor digitorum communis and flexor sublimus and profundus).

In a T_1 lesion, all hand muscles function, but with partial paralysis of the adductor pollicis, interossi, and lumbricals, and paralysis of the abductor pollicis brevis. Sensory loss occurs on the ulnar side of the forearm from the wrist to the elbow.

RADIAL NERVE

The radial nerve arises from C_5, C_6, C_7, C_8, and T_1 as a continuation of the posterior cord in the axilla (Fig. 2–40). In the upper arm it winds around the humerus in a spiral groove that passes posteriorly from the medial to the lateral aspect of the arm. It enters the forearm in front of the lateral epicondyle, between the brachialis and the brachioradialis muscles, which it supplies.

In the upper forearm it divides into two branches:

1. The posterior interosseous nerve branch (purely motor).
2. A continuation of the nerve into the superficial branch (sensory).

The posterior interosseous nerve supplies the following muscles:

1. Supinator $(C_5–C_8)$, which supinates the forearm (Fig. 2–41).
2. Anconeus
3. Extensor digitorum communis (C_7, C_8) (Fig. 2–42).
4. Extensor digiti quinti proprius (C_7, C_8).
5. Extensor carpi radialis and ulnaris (C_7, C_8) (Fig. 2–43).
6. Abductor pollicis longus (C_7, C_8) (Fig. 2–44).
7. Extensor pollicis longus (see Fig. 2–44 above) and brevis $(C_7, C_8$; Fig. 2–45).

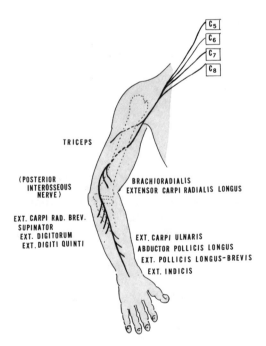

Figure 2–40. Radial nerve.

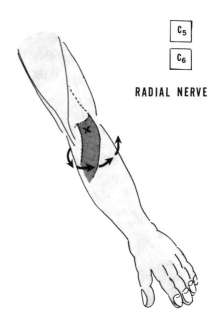

C_5

C_6

RADIAL NERVE

Figure 2–41. Supinator. The supinator is supplied by the radial nerve and roots of C_5 and C_6. It supinates the forearm, and is a deep muscle of the forearm extensor group originating from the lateral epicondyle of the humerus. The supinator inserts upon the dorsal lateral surfaces of the upper third of the radius.

The superficial branch, which is a continuation of the radial nerve, supplies the sensation of the dorsum of the hand (Fig. 2–46).

SUMMARY OF NERVE LESIONS

Below is a summary of the nerves whose lesions can be tested and diagnosed.

Median Nerve

This innervates the flexor carpi radialis, flexor digitorum profundus of the index finger, flexor pollicis longus, flexor digitorum superficialis, and the abductor pollicis brevis.

Figure 2–42. Extensor digitorum communis (and extensor digiti quinti proprius). It originates from the lateral epicondyle of the humerus (see Fig. 1–53) and inserts into the proximal dorsal aspect of the middle phalanx

RADIAL NERVE

(EXAMINER)

C_7

C_8

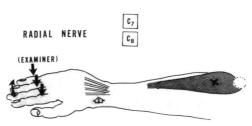

and distal phalanx (see Fig. 1–72). As the examiner resists, the patient attempts to extend all four fingers (index to little: 2, 3, 4, 5).

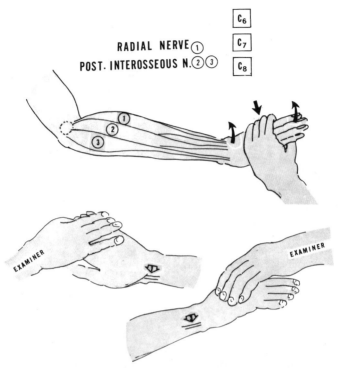

Figure 2–43. Extensor carpi radialis, extensor digitorum communis, and extensor carpi ulnaris. All these muscles originate from the epicondylar area of the humerus. (1) The extensor carpi radialis attaches with the brevis to the bases of the second and third metacarpals (see Fig. 1–53). They are pure wrist muscles and dorsiflex the wrist in a radial direction. (2) The extensor digitorum communis is depicted in Fig. 2–42. (3) The extensor carpi ulnaris originates from the lateral epicondyle of the humerus and inserts upon the dorsal surface of the fifth metacarpal. It dorsiflexes the wrist in an ulnar direction.

Severence of the **MEDIAN** nerve causes the following:

1. Hypesthesia of the palmar area (Fig. 2–47). Total anesthesia occurs usually only on the palmar and dorsal aspects of the terminal phalanges of the index and middle fingers.
2. Weakness of the wrist flexors and pronation of the forearm.
3. Inability to flex the thumb, and the index and middle fingers.
4. Difficulty in opposing the tip of the thumb to the tip of the other fingers.
5. Slight hyperextension of the first and middle fingers at the metacarpophalangeal joints.

Figure 2–44. Abductor pollicis longus and extensor pollicis longus. The abductor pollicis longus (1) originates from the dorsal surface of the ulna, the radius, and the interosseous membrane. It inserts upon the latter aspect of the base of the first metacarpal. The extensor pollicis longus (2) originates from the middle third of the ulnar shaft (below the abductor pollicis longus) and inserts upon the dorsal aspect of the base of the terminal phalanx of the thumb. Both muscles are innervated by the posterior interosseous nerve roots C_7 and C_8.

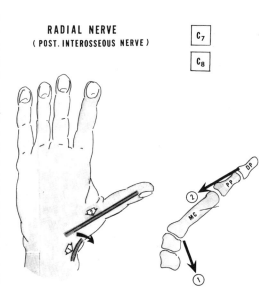

6. Functional loss of precision grip, with resulting difficulty in picking up small objects or identifying small objects when blindfolded.
7. Weakened power grip due to failure of thumb stabilization.

Figure 2–45. Extensor pollicis brevis and extensor indicis proprius. The extensor pollicis brevis (EPB) originates from the shaft of the radius and inserts upon the dorsal aspect of the first phalanx of the thumb. Its action is to abduct and extend the base of the thumb. The extensor indicis proprius (EIP) originates from the lower half of the ulna and inserts into the tendon of the extensor digitorum communis to extend the index finger. Both muscles are innervated by the radial nerve with roots C_7 and C_8.

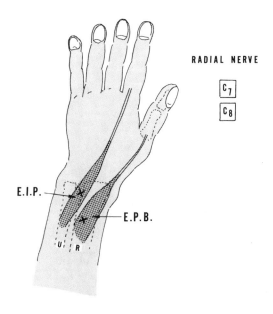

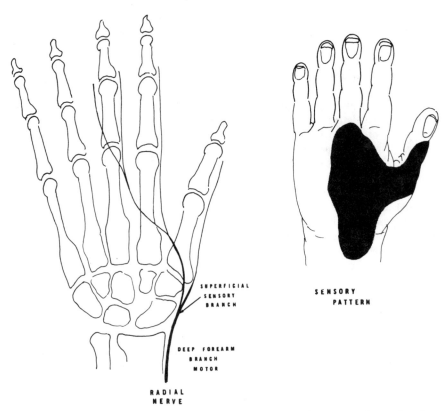

Figure 2–46. Radial nerve. The sensory pattern is shown on the right, the motor distribution on the left. Above the elbow, the nerve supplies the elbow extensor (triceps), flexion (brachioradialis), and the extensor carpi radialis. Below the elbow the nerve supplies extension of the wrist in the ulnar deviation, extension of the fingers, and extension of the distal phalanx of the thumb and index finger.

Ulnar Nerve

Severence of the ULNAR nerve causes the following:

1. Hypesthesia of the ulnar aspect of the hand.
2. Inability to flex the distal phalanges of the fourth and fifth fingers.
3. Loss of ulnar wrist flexion.
4. Inability to hold paper between the thumb and index finger.
5. Weakness in spreading the fingers.

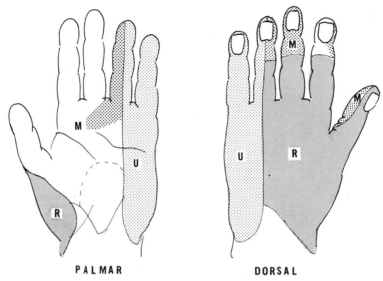

PALMAR   DORSAL

Figure 2-47. Sensory mapping of peripheral nerves. The schematic areas of sensory innervation of the median nerve (M), radial nerve (R), and ulnar (U) are shown. The dorsum of the hand is variable and the radial nerve may have *no* sensory area or merely a small area over the first dorsal interosseous.

6. Difficulty in forming a perfect letter *O* with the thumb and index finger.
7. Hyperextension (30°) of the ring and little fingers at the metacarpophalangeal joints.
8. Functional difficulty in writing, as a result of loss of sensation of the little finger, poor pinch grip, and loss of thumb adduction. Power grip is lost due to weakness of the finger flexors.
9. Severence of the ulnar nerve at the elbow causes flexion deformity of the fourth and fifth fingers, hypothenar eminence atrophy, atrophy of the interossei, and atrophy of the web between the thumb and index finger.

Radial Nerve

Severence of the **RADIAL** nerve causes the following:

1. Pronation of the hand.
2. Flexion of the elbow and inability to extend the hand (Fig. 2-48).

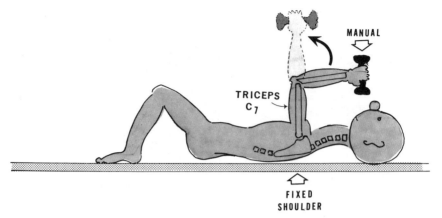

MANUAL

TRICEPS
C₇

FIXED
SHOULDER

Figure 2–48. Muscle examination of triceps (C_7). With patient supine and arm held vertically, the triceps can more easily be tested for strength and for endurance. In this position the scapular muscles are fixed, allowing the triceps to be isolated (C_7). Fatigue may indicate a C_7 lesion when a single effort fails to reveal weakness.

3. Wrist "drop."
4. Inability to extend the proximal phalanges.
5. Inability to extend or abduct the thumb.
6. Hypesthesia of the dorsum of the hand, although there may be NO sensory loss.
7. Absence of the brachioradialis reflex (Fig. 2–49) and possible absence or diminution of the triceps reflex.
8. A lesion of the radial nerve at the upper humerus will affect the triceps. With a lesion at the lower humerus, the brachioradialis and extensor carpi radialis longus will be affected, with possible sparing of the triceps.

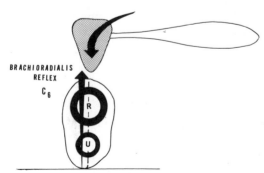

BRACHIORADIALIS
REFLEX

C₆

R

U

Figure 2–49. Brachioradialis reflex test. With the forearm gently supported and neutral between pronation and supination, a gentle tap on the distal radius or the styloid (attachment of the brachioradialis muscle) will cause reflex flexion of the elbow. The fingers may also flex but are not a part of the brachioradialis reflex. Finger flexion with no elbow flexion—an *inversion*—implies a C_6 lesion.

MANAGEMENT OF NERVE INJURIES

Nerve response to injury proceeds in two phases.[18] The first phase is disintegration of the axon, with a breakdown of its myelin sheath (wallerian degeneration). The basement membranes surrounding the Schwann cells (Fig. 2–50) persist during wallerian degeneration and form tubes, within which the Schwann cells proliferate to give rise to longitudinal columns.[19] The end receptors also undergo degeneration.

The second phase is neuronal regeneration, with growth of the axon in the direction of the remaining distal endoneural tube (Fig. 2–51). If the injury has not led to nerve cell death, the axon will regenerate. Nerve regeneration occurs by outgrowth of the proximal stump and not by autoregeneration of the degenerated distal nerve.[20] After a latency period of 24 hours, the cut axon tip bulges into a growth cone. Growth of this tip proceeds with spouting of collaterals. There is also a proliferation of the nodes of Ranvier proximal to the axon tip.

After bridging the gap at the site of injury the axonal spouts grow down the distal tube (by 4–5 days postinjury) at a reported growth of 8.5 mm per day.[21]

After 24 hours a few of the spouts have reached the area of injury. New Schwann cells also develop.[22] The distal axon undergoes wallerian degeneration and the remaining debris is removed by the now phagocytotic action of the remaining Schwann cells. These Schwann cells proliferate within the remaining basal laminar tubes of the distal nerve and form longitudinal rows that can accept the regenerating proximal axon. The regenerating axons do not permeate the old Schwann tubes but create new tubes as they penetrate the longitudinal rows of Schwann cells.

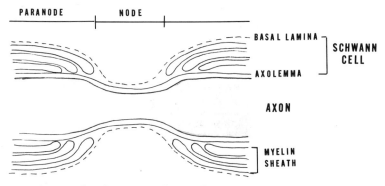

Figure 2–50. A node of Ranvier. The myelinated axon is narrowed at each node of Ranvier formed by Schwann cells that invaginate to form a node with the remaining portion being a paranode.

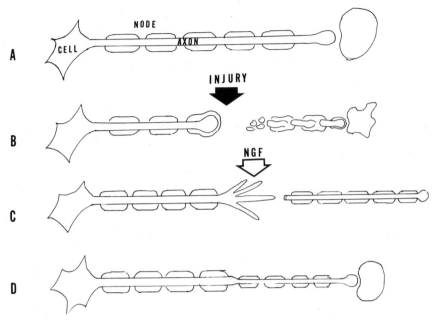

Figure 2–51. Nerve regeneration. *(A)* Depicts a normal nerve with intact cell body, a continuous axon and nodes (of Ranvier) and the end organ acting upon the end organ. *(B)* Injury causing degeneration of the distal axon, myelin, nodes and end organ. *(C)* Depicts distal nerve filaments leaving the proximal segment "in search of" the distal segment aided by nerve growth factor (NGF). *(D)* Union of the severed segments with the distal axon, node as yet immature.

Regeneration has been postulated to occur at a rate of 1 to 3 mm per day, after a latency period of 3 to 4 weeks. After bridging the gap (usually by 4–5 days postinjury), the axonal sprouts allegedly grow at the rate of 8.5 mm per day in the arm and 1.5 mm in the hand.[23] A nerve growth factor is essential in this regenerative process.

The growth of regenerating nerves may be influenced by unfavorable factors such as scarring at the injury site; short circuiting of the spouting axons; mismatching of the motor, sensory, or sympathetic fibers; and total degeneration of the end organs, either sensory or motor.

REHABILITATION PRINCIPLES

Acute Phase

The objectives to be met here are protection of the injured nerve, and prevention of joint contracture and subsequent injury to the anesthetized finger(s).[24] Care to ensure proper wound healing is mandatory. There are on the market today many pharmacological agents that are advocated for application to the wound site to insure proper healing of the wound and prevention of scarring, as well as infection. None are without potentially detrimental side effects.

Wound healing is a dynamic coordinated effort to ensure cell multiplication and active migration of normal tissues: collagen, and nerve and blood vessels.[25] Initially the intent is to minimize the inflammatory phase by cleansing the wound of debris, invading bacteria, and unwanted chemicals. Ultimately, encouragement of the proper fibroplasia, which begins 2 to 6 weeks postinjury, is indicated. The final stage of healing is formation of scar, which must be guided in its maturation and remodeling activity.[26]

Postinjury or postoperative immobilization (splinting) minimizes the tension at the injury or repair site, protects the nerve from further disruption, and allows resolution of the inflammation. Splints, either static or dynamic, are addressed in Chapter 10.

The aim of postimmobilization treatment is to recover the range of motion lost or impaired during the period of immobilization. The initiation of passive or active assisted exercises depends upon the patient's progress and the site of joint involvement. Both motor and sensory functional retraining are essential in hand rehabilitation, and constitute the educational aspect of rehabilitation.

Electrical Stimulation

Electrical stimulation has been advocated to reduce pain, increase muscle contraction to counteract atrophy from neuromuscular dysfunction, and enhance tissue healing.[27] It also has been advocated in neuromuscular "reeducation." Its value as a muscle strengthener for disuse atrophy has had varying justification for decades. It has been advocated for use in patients who have no or limited voluntary use of an impaired muscle,[28,29] but most studies conclude that electrical stimulation superimposed upon voluntary exercise gives the same result as voluntary exercise alone. Reinervation of muscles is not influenced by electrical stimulation.[30]

NERVE COMPRESSION SYNDROMES

Nerve compression, considered a "neuropraxia," is a conduction (nerve) block that has been experimentally reproduced in animals by the application of a tourniquet in an effort to clarify what happens in humans. Neuropraxia has also been considered as a conduction block that causes muscle weakness without significant atrophy and usually spares sensation.[30,31]

In the laboratory a controlled pneumatic tourniquet application that controls the site, duration, and extent of nerve compression has been used. Ochoa and colleagues applied a tourniquet to a baboon hind leg and found evidence of longitudinal displacement of the nodes of Ranvier (see Fig. 2–50) to a significant degree, most prominently under the proximal edge of the cuff (Fig. 2–52).[32]

The fact that motor impairment has been noted clinically when there is electrical evidence of denervation without nerve conduction delay suggests that "axonotomesis occurs without coincident neuropraxia." This fact may explain why patients with carpal tunnel nerve compression syndrome occasionally have EMG (electromyographic) evidence of thenar muscle denervation without prolonged distal motor or sensory latencies.[33]

These tourniquet studies are suggestive of the pathology in most nerve compression syndromes, except that the pressures exceed the force and duration clinically noted or even possible in man. In tourniquet injury, mast cells have been found in edema with increased vascular permeability. This may explain the pathology of compression syndromes: intraneural edema and microvessel obliteration, which causes ischemia of the axon and subsequent degeneration.

Fortunately tissues so damaged have shown the ability to recover, although not spontaneously or rapidly. The myelin disruption (neuropraxia) accounts for the nerve conduction block, which recovers after some months. The time required for recovery is related to the number of Ranvier nodes involved. In many cases, sensory modalities of crude

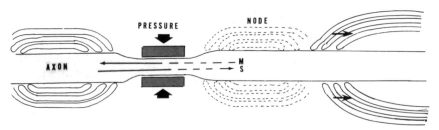

Figure 2–52. Tourniquet-induced nerve degeneration. Application of a tourniquet upon a myelinated peripheral nerve causes a longitudinal displacement of the nodes of Ranvier especially at the proximal edge of the tourniquet (pressure). The dotted figure is the normal site of the node prior to pressure and the node with arrows show the migration. The pressure upon the axon causes nerve conduction deficit on the sensory (S) and motor (M) nerves (arrows).

and light touch and pinprick are spared, whereas careful mapping with vibration and two-point discrimination reveals evidence of subtle sensory loss.

Carpal Tunnel Syndrome

Carpal tunnel syndrome (CTS) is currently a frequent source of pain, impairment, and disability, whereas it was rarely diagnosed 50 years ago.[34] This is probably due to a greater awareness of its presence and the availability of more precise diagnostic procedures which confirm the diagnosis suggested by its clinical manifestations. This syndrome is a median nerve compression syndrome and thus is discussed later in this chapter in the section on nerve control of the hand.

The contents of the carpal tunnel are depicted in Fig. 2–53.

Carpal tunnel syndrome was originally described by Phalen,[35] and was considered as a diagnosis in persons complaining of pain and paresthesias of the thumb, index finger, long finger, and the radial half of the ring finger: that is, the dermatome area of the median nerve.

This condition was previously found to occur predominantly in middle-aged women and to manifest itself as a nocturnal occurrence. Currently there is another population that is becoming afflicted and which includes persons of either sex whose occupation leads to "repeti-

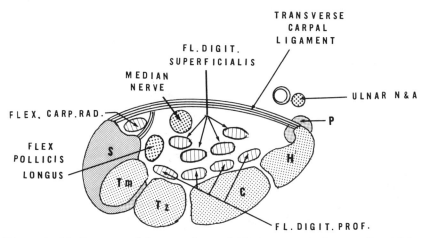

Figure 2–53. Contents of the carpal tunnel. The concave palmar surface of the carpal rows is crossed by the transverse carpal ligament. The tunnel contains the median nerve and all the flexor tendons and their sheaths. Thickening of the tendon sheaths, the carpal ligament, or deformation of the bony structure can compress the median nerve.

tive injuries," which are allegedly sustained in the work situation. Occupations where this syndrome occurs are those that involve repetitive actions involving flexion-extension of the wrist, a strong gripping action, and even exposure to vibration.[36]

Initially the CTS syndrome presents as a sensory manifestation of pain, tingling, and numbness, with the distribution noted above. Loss of sensation, motor weakness, loss of coordination, and atrophy are later symptoms.

The syndrome is classified as acute or chronic. The "acute" syndrome is relatively rare, a sequela of trauma, and is characterized by rapid development of intense symptoms. A less "acute" form is more insidious and initially less intense. The need for awareness of this 'acute' type is that it incurs from the same pathophysiology but demands more acute decompression to prevent permanent residual damage. It is often difficult to differentiate an acute carpal tunnel syndrome from acute median nerve trauma.

Chronic carpal tunnel syndrome is usually gradual in its onset and initially involves one finger. As it progresses, other fingers are usually involved, and ultimately all fingers innervated by the median nerve may be affected.

Symptoms are variable. Typically they occur at night, but they may occur after repetitive manual activity.[37] The symptoms and ultimate pathology of median nerve compression in CTS are due to alterations of fluid pressures and dynamics that lead to ischemic changes of the nerve.[38,39] (See Fig. 2–54.)

In early CTS cases, studies reveal that prolongation of sensory latencies occurs earlier than prolongation of motor latencies. Gross morphological studies of the nerve at this stage reveal little or no significant alterations; thus, full recovery can be expected with early recognition and attention.

At a later stage in CTS, the sensory changes remain constant and motor deficit becomes noted. At this point, full recovery may not be attainable. In advanced (chronic) stages, sensory and motor loss is noted, atrophy of the involved muscles is apparent, and the median nerve exhibits demyelination and fibrosis. Even now surgical decompression may afford partial relief, but total recovery is doubtful.

The muscles involved are those of the thumb (opponens pollicis, abductor pollicis brevis, and the first and second lumbrical muscles). In testing, it is necessary to be aware of the function of these muscles:

1. Abductor pollicis brevis elevates the thumb at a right angle to the plane of the palm. This action is an unreliable test of median nerve function, however, as this movement can be performed by combined action of the flexor pollicis brevis (ulnar nerve) and the abductor pollicis longus (radial nerve).

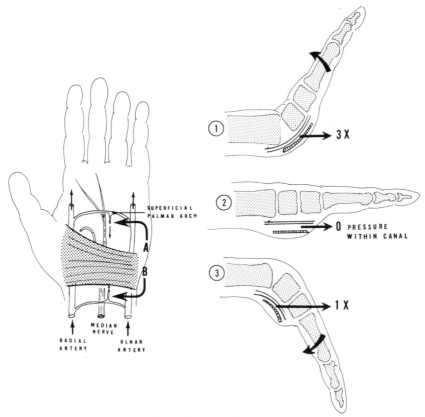

Figure 2–54. Mechanism of parethesiae of carpal tunnel syndrome. The large figure shows the arterial circulation of the median nerve receiving a small branch distally from the superficial palmar arch (A) and a branch proximally from the ulnar artery (B). Compression can occur distally from occupational pressures on the palm and proximally from prolonged flexion or extension of the wrist with simultaneous finger flexion compressing the small proximal arterial branch. (1) Wrist extension (dorsiflexion), which creates three times the pressure within the carpal tunnel as is found during wrist flexion (3). During extension (2) there is release of the arterial compression.

    2. Opponens pollicis approximates the tip of the thumb to the tip of the little finger. This movement can be mimicked by the flexor pollicis brevis and the adductor pollicis, both of which are innervated by the ulnar nerve.

    3. The first and second lumbrical muscles extend the fingers at the interphalangeal joint with the metacarpophalangeal joint hyperextended. This action can be mimicked by the extensor communis digitorium when extension of the metacarpophalangeal joint is eliminated.

4. Flexor pollicis brevis has a dual innervation (median and ulnar); thus its action is also unreliable in testing for CTS.

It is apparent that precise motor testing to ascertain median nerve function is precarious, and that misinterpretation is possible. Also, the usual innervation of the median nerve may be confusing, as when there exists an "all-median-nerve hand," where the entire hand is supplied by the median nerve with no ulnar innervation. An "all-ulnar-hand" may exist. These variants can be ascertained by EMG studies with percutaneous electrical stimulation.

Diagnosis of CTS must establish that there is objective median nerve compression. Numerous tests have been established:

Phalen's Test: Holding the wrist at a full flexed position causes paresthesia (numbness and tingling) of the fingers on the radial side of the hand (median dermatome).

Tinel's Sign. Percussion of the median nerve at the wrist reproduces the tingling in the involved fingers.

A recent review article evaluated the value of Phalen's test and the Tinel sign test and concluded that the former was reliable and the latter was not.[40] Tinel first described a tingling sensation, which he noted when the proximal stump of an injured nerve was percussed, and considered this an indication of regeneration.[41]

When carpal tunnel median nerve syndrome was first described the Tinel sign was not mentioned.[42] Phalen mentioned the Tinel sign in 1950 and claimed that percussion of the median nerve below the transverse carpal ligament was a confirmatory sign.[43]

The exact technique for eliciting a Tinel sign was not defined and varied from "gentle tapping over the median nerve" to "light percussion."[44] A sharp blow over the normal median nerve can cause tingling.[45] The number of taps as well as the force remains unspecified, and review of the literature leads to the conclusion that the Phalen test remains more predictable and the Tinel sign of little value.

Drawing of Area of Paresthesia. The patient can draw on the palmar surface of the hand the area where paresthesias are observed.

Two-Point Discrimination. The patient may be unable to discriminate two stimuli which are more than 6 mm apart.

Inflation Testing. Inflating a sphygmomanometer cuff around the forearm, or manually compressing the radial and ulnar arteries, may cause an unpleasant tingling and numbness of the hand. Release of this pressure results in persistence of a "pins and needles" sensation for 5 to 10 seconds.

*Distal Sensory Latency Velocity.** An orthodromic stimulus recorded across the wrist revealing prolongation beyond 3.5 mm/sec.

*Distal Motor Latency Velocity.** Orthodromic stimulus and recording across the wrist becoming diagnostic when latencies are greater than 4.5 mm/sec.

*Electromyography (EMG).** This may be used to determine denervation of the thenar muscles. Positive when there has been further nerve compression with nerve impairment.

The causes of CTS are many, and may include one or more of the following:

1. Repetitive trauma.
2. Exposure to excessive vibration.
3. Unusual immobilization with the wrist in an ulnar deviated position following a Colle's fracture.
4. Structural (bony) alteration of the carpal canal.
5. Abnormal inclusions, such as osteophytes, lipomas, and so on, within the canal.
6. Neuropathic medical conditions, such as diabetes, alcoholism, rheumatoid arthritis, gout, and so on.
7. Abnormal fluid balance from pregnancy, myxedema, Raynaud's disease, and so forth.

Besides a careful mechanical evaluation after a precise medical history, radiological studies can be performed to determine the competence of the canal.

Conservative Management. Alteration of the daily working factors which are considered as causative and splinting the wrist in a neutral position during the day AND night for several weeks are valid measures. Oral anti-inflammatory medication also has value. Injection of steroids into the carpal tunnel affords benefits that are often transient unless the injection is given early in the condition, when the effects may last longer.[46]

When there is no or minimal response to conservative management, decompression of the nerve is indicated. Surgery may be via endoscopic or open procedures.

It must be noted that there are numerous anatomical variations of the median nerve at the wrist.[47] The variations may be classified as (1) motor branch anomalies, (2) multiple divisions of the nerve, (3) neural

---

*Diagnostic test done by an electromyographer when the clinical condition has been suspected following a careful history and a positive Phalen and Tinel test. Other tests are available but not imperative.

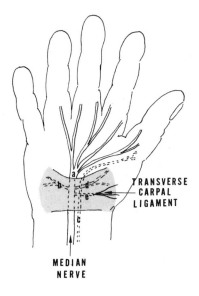

Figure 2–55. Anatomical variations of the median nerve at the wrist. (A) The usual position and distribution of the median nerve. (B) A transligamentous distribution to the abductor digiti quinti. (C) A divided median nerve. (D) Transligamentous course that remains under the ligament. (E) The transligamentous course where the nerve penetrates the ligament.

loops, and (4) aberrant muscles. The course of the recurrent motor branch in relation to the transverse carpal ligament may (a) run distal to the ligament (extraligamentous), (b) be within the tunnel (subligamentous), (c) pierce the ligament (transligamentous), or (d) travel within the substance of the ligament (intraligamentous) (Fig. 2–55). The tremendous variations in the motor branch of the median nerve require great caution on the part of the surgeon operating on this syndrome.[48] Visualization of the nerve branches must be assured in the surgical release of compression.[49–51]

The endoscopic approach to decompression decreases postoperative pain and results in less scarring, more rapid recovery, and less loss of grip pain. Visibility is poor in this approach, and there is difficulty in controlling bleeding, hence only a surgeon with vast experience should undertake this approach.

The short incision distal to the palm, avoiding the palmar sensory branch of the median nerve allegedly causes less postoperative morbidity[52] and better cosmesis.[53] The diminished visibility available to the surgeon may result in missing the frequent variants of median nerve.[54]

It is essential that a surgeon have formal training and cadaver practice before undertaking this procedure. The duration of surgical time is the same as for the open approach, but there is need of special equipment, which costs between $5000 and $10,000 with optical accessories and electronics in place.

The technique of endoscopic surgery merits discussion even though this text is not surgical. Choosing the site of incision for insertion of the

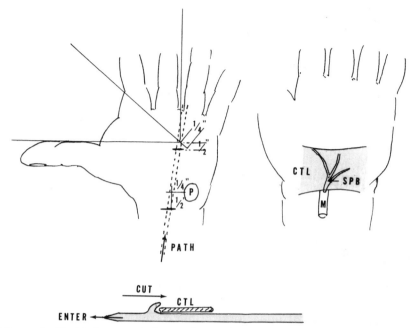

Figure 2–56. Endoscopic release of carpal tunnel syndrome (ERCT). Upper left: The site of entry of the trocar is measured by palpating the pisiform bone (P) and measuring medially ¼ inch then proximally ½ inch. The second site at the trocar exits is in the distal palm as indicated. The path of the trocar is between these two sites. Upper right: The presence of the sensory palmar branch (SPB) of the median nerve (M) is shown superficial to the carpal transverse ligament (CTL). Lower: Upon removal of the trocar the arthroscope is inserted in the same path. After passing the carpal transverse ligament (CTL) it is slowly removed causing the cutting knife blade to cut the ligament.

instrument requires palpating the pisiform bone (see Fig. 1–38), which is used as the reference for determining the points of entry and exit (Fig. 2–56). After entry of the trocar through the incision ¼ inch medial and ½ inch distal to the pisiform bone, the trocar exits in the distal palm, and the cutting instrument can be inserted along the path of the trocar from the proximal to the distal insertion. When the instrument is removed, it severs the transverse carpal ligament.

An incision to admit the entrance of a trocar is usually small and avoids the sensory branch of the median nerve to the palm; this branch often complicates carpal tunnel release surgery.

Endoscopic carpal tunnel release (ECTR) is not for everyone.[55] It should not be considered for patients who have had prior carpal tunnel surgery or for patients with systemic problems that have caused or contributed to their tenosynovitis.

The alleged benefit of endoscopic versus open release of the carpal tunnel is a more rapid return to employment with the former, a factor which translates into monetary terms.[56] There is also allegedly less palmar sensory deficit.

Recovery of function and loss of pain and paresthesia after surgical decompression has not been well documented in long-term follow-up studies. In a recent study, 93 patients under the age of 55 were followed up 2 years after surgical decompression.[57] Thirty-eight patients had symptoms similar to those they had prior to surgery, with 12 patients unable to resume their preoperative occupation. These studies also revealed that most patients who had a continuation of symptoms and disability had returned to the occupations requiring repetitive hand and arm movements that were considered to be causative of the condition originally.[58,59]

Normally the strength of the dominant and the nondominant hand does not differ significantly.[60] In CTS, there is relative weakness of the impaired hand, which persists after surgery unless efforts at regaining strength and endurance are invoked.[61] Rehabilitation of these patients may also demand modification of the resumed occupation.[62]

Synovectomy. At open surgical intervention, the surgeon finds a flexor tendon synovitis, often which has caused or contributed to carpal tunnel syndrome. If this synovitis is secondary to the nerve compression, it will subside by mere decompression. If the synovitis is a concurrent disease entity, such as rheumatoid arthritis or a variant, synovectomy may be indicated.

If severe fibrotic changes are found at the time of the tunnel decompression, interfascicular neurolysis may be valuable in restoring normal neural flow.[54]

As the transverse carpal ligament is a proximal pully of the finger flexors, its division may impair the biomechanics of flexor function after release.[63] In this case, reconstruction of the transverse carpal ligament is indicated.

Postoperative care has usually invoked immobilization, and presents rehabilitation problems that allegedly are absent with endoscopic surgery.

Pronator Teres Median Nerve Compression

The median nerve leaves the cubital fossa, passing between the heads of the pronator teres muscle, it then passes under the tendinous edge of the flexor digitorum sublimis muscle (Fig. 2–57). Its course through the pronator teres muscle varies. It may be between the heads (56%), behind the heads (11%), through the humeral head (3%), and

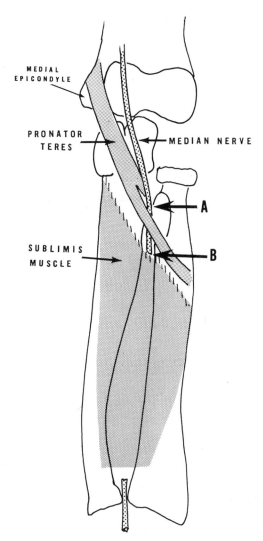

Figure 2–57. Pronator teres median nerve compression. The median nerve leaves the cubital fossa passing between the heads of the pronator teres muscle then passes under the tendinous edge of the flexor digitorum sublimis muscle. Upon leaving the pronator teres the median nerve gives rise to the anterior interroseous nerve.

through the ulnar head (2%).[64] In some cases the ulnar head of the pronator teres is missing. Upon leaving the pronator teres the median nerve gives rise to the anterior interrosseous nerve.

After traversing the teres muscle, the median nerve divides under the tendinous arch of the flexor digitorum sublimis (FDS) and into the layer between the FDS and the flexor digitorum profundus (FDP). It runs between the FDS and the FDP, and ultimately between the flexor carpi radialis (FCR) and the flexor palmaris longus (FPL), to reach the carpal tunnel.

In the forearm, the median nerve supplies the pronator teres, flexor carpi radialis, palmaris longus, and digitorum superficialis. Just distal to the pronator muscle, the median nerve sends branches to the ulnar half of the flexor digitorum profundus, flexor pollicis longus, and pronator quadratus. This anatomic knowledge is vital in diagnostically exploring the muscles involved in this syndrome.

The pronator teres pronates the forearm with the elbow bent, preventing rotation by elimination of pronation from the brachioradialis and the long flexors of the forearm.

There are numerous causes of nerve compression, varying from direct trauma,[65] static compression from a fibrous band, and prolonged external compression, as in "honeymoon paralysis."[66]

Symptoms and Signs. Subjective symptoms and objective signs of median nerve involvement in the upper extremity are similar to those of carpal tunnel syndrome, except that the pronator teres syndrome not only involves the muscles of the thenar eminence but also the flexors of the wrist and the fingers. The patient's complaints are related to the thumb, index finger, and middle finger flexion. Sensory disturbances involve the volar and dorsal surfaces of the hand, palm, and several fingers.[67]

Sensory disturbances of the palm indicate compression "proximal" to the tunnel, as the median nerve normally gives off the palmaris branch prior to entering the tunnel. This fact is probably the most important diagnostic sign differentiating the pronator teres syndrome from carpal tunnel median nerve compression.

A stress test result that suggests pronator teres compression is the evoking of pain and paresthesia by "resisted pronation of the forearm with the elbow extended."[68] Further aggravation of the symptoms occurs on resistance of flexion of the elbow and simultaneous supination of the forearm, and implicates the lacertus fibrosus. Resistance of flexion of the proximal interphalangeal joint of the middle finger implicates the FDS muscle belly.

A positive Tinel's sign can be elicited by tapping or exerting direct pressure in the region of the two heads of the pronator teres muscle below the cubital space.

Electromyographic studies assist in diagnosis by demonstrating abnormalities and delayed conduction velocity of the FCR, FDS, and FPL. In contrast to carpal tunnel median nerve compression, which usually involves the muscles of the thenar eminence, compression at the pronator teres site involves not only the thenar muscles but also those of the wrist and finger flexors.

As the median nerve gives off a palmar branch before entering the carpal tunnel, a sensory deficit of the palm implies median nerve compression proximal to the carpal tunnel.

Treatment of Pronator Teres Syndrome. Most pronator teres syndromes (PTS) are mild and self-limited; thus merely reducing provocative movement of the forearm, wrist, and finger flexors for several weeks will be beneficial. This can be assisted by splinting the forearm in a neutral position between pronation and supination. Local injection of steroids into the region of compression is also valuable.[69]

Persistence of symptoms and objective evidence of insidious paresis and anasthesia justify surgical decompression. This allows identification of the involved structures, release of the origin of the humeral head of the pronator, and even neurolysis of the median nerve if indicated by persistence of symptoms.[70]

Anterior Interosseous Syndrome

The motor branch of the median nerve, the anterior interosseous nerve, can undergo compression in the cubital region and result in impaired function of the distal phalanges of the thumb and index finger.

The anterior interosseous nerve originates from the division of the median nerve, and progresses under the deep fascial layer of the flexor digitorum superficialis running along the interosseous membrane. It ultimately innervates the flexor pollicis longus and the flexor digitorum profundus to the second finger. There are many variations in the course of this nerve, with the result that many authors consider this syndrome to be identical to the pronator teres syndrome.[71]

As numerous fascial tunnels may exist in the forearm, which tunnel is involved in this syndrome remains unresolved.

Clinically the patient develops an inabilty to pinch between the thumb and index finger due to paresis of the distal phalanges of both fingers. Pinching is attempted with both joints remaining extended. In addition, the patient is unable to clench the fist or write (Fig. 2–58).

Treatment consists of immobilization and avoidance of the discovered causative factors, but when there is persistence of symptoms and EMG verification, surgical decompression is indicated.

Ulnar Nerve Compression

The ulnar nerve is subjected to compression at numerous sites along its course. At the wrist, the ulnar nerve enters the hand in a shallow trough between the pisiform bone and the hook of the hamate bone (Guyon's canal) (Fig. 2–59).[72] The floor of this "tunnel" is a thin

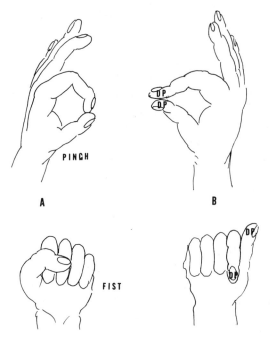

Figure 2-58. Anterior interosseous syndrome. The motor deficit of the anterior interosseous nerve syndrome causes inability to flex the distal phalanges (DP) of the index finger and thumb. The normal pinch (*upper A*) with tip to tip opposition is not possible (*upper B*) with the distal phalanges extended. In making a fist (*lower A*) the normally flexed fingers cannot flex at the index and thumb distal phalanges (*lower B*).

layer of ligament and muscle. Its roof is the volar carpal ligament and the palmaris longus muscle (Fig. 2-60). Proximal to its entry, the nerve divides into a dorsal branch and a palmar branch; the latter further divides into superficial and deep palmar branches that run into the tunnel. Only these two terminal branches run into the tunnel; therefore compression due to tunnel entrapment spares the dorsal branch.

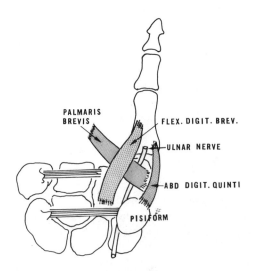

Figure 2-59. Ulnar nerve entry into hand at wrist (Guyon's canal).

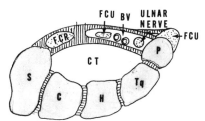

Figure 2–60. Guyon's canal (ulnar nerve tunnel). The ulnar nerve canal (Guyon's) is adjacent to the carpal tunnel (CT) but its contents are subject to different pressures. Guyon's canal is within the flexor retinaculum, which contains the ulnar nerve, flexor carpi ulnaris tendinous insert (FCU) and blood vessels (the ulnar artery and vein) (BV) and the flexor carpii radialis muscle (FCR). The base of the carpal tunnel contains the scaphoid (navicular) (S), capitate (C), hamate (H), triquetrium (Tq) and pisiform (P) bones.

The superficial branch of the palmar branch innervates the palmaris brevis muscle, the palmar skin of the fifth finger, and the ulnar skin of the fourth finger. The deep branch innervates the hypothenar muscles, the two lateral lumbricals, all the interosseous muscles, the adductor pollicis, and the deep head of the flexor pollicis brevis muscles. Compression of the superficial branch causes motor and sensory symptoms (see Figs. 2–36 and 2–37), whereas compression of the deep branch causes only motor symptoms.[73]

Just as there are many variations in the division of the median nerve at the wrist and the hand, there are many variations of the ulnar nerve (Fig. 2–61).[73]

There are numerous etiologies to ulnar nerve compression at Guyon's canal but most are traumatic and result from such activities as bicycle or motor cycle riding, operating a pneumatic drill, and so on. Ganglions secondary to degenerative arthritis, giant tumors of the tendon sheaths, and so on have been described.[74]

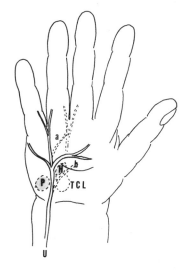

Figure 2–61. Variations of the ulnar nerve. The normal branching of the ulnar nerve (U) may have variations. After passing the pisiform bone (P) and the hook of the hamate (H) there can be a communicating branch between the fourth and third digital nerves (a) the nerve may divide around the hook (b) or around the tendon of the flexor carpi ulnaris (not shown). Numerous accessory muscles (of the flexor digiti minimi, abductor digiti minimi or palmaris) may exist requiring accessory nerves.

Patients may describe "difficulty" in hand-grasping activities and paresthesia of the dermatomal regions of the ulnar nerve. Motor weakness may be described as "clumsiness" in performing fine movements, and loss of "pinch" strength of the thumb may also be apparent. Atrophy of the interossei gradually becomes apparent, with deepening of the interosseous grooves on the dorsum of the hand. Tinel's sign over the ulnar nerve may be elicited. Confirmation by EMG is diagnostic.[75] Special radiological studies will reveal anatomical variations in the canal.[76]

Treatment should be conservative: avoiding the activities found to be responsible, oral anti-inflammatory medication, steroid injection, and splinting. If there is not significant relief, surgery is advocated before 6 months have passed.[77] If both syndromes (Guyon's and carpal tunnel) are present, a release of the median nerve should also be contemplated.[78]

Piso-Hamate Hiatus Syndrome

The syndrome is due to compression of the deep branch of the ulnar nerve as it passes through a fibro-osseous tunnel formed by the tendinous origin of the hypothenar muscles (Fig. 2–62). This syndrome is similar to the previous syndrome (Guyon's syndrome) except that only a motor branch is compressed. This condition is also known as Uriburu[79] or the piso-hamate hiatus syndrome. Since this syndrome affects the nerve branch before it enters the tendinous arch, it does not affect the abductor digiti quinti minimi muscle.

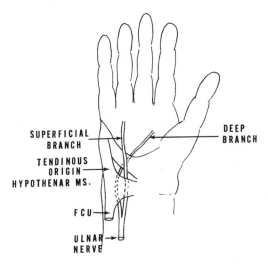

SUPERFICIAL BRANCH

DEEP BRANCH

TENDINOUS ORIGIN HYPOTHENAR MS.

FCU

ULNAR NERVE

Figure 2–62. Syndrome of the deep branch of the ulnar nerve. This syndrome is otherwise termed the Piso-Hamate Hiatus Syndrome with the FCU being the flexor carpi ulnaris. The branches pass under the tendinous arch of the palm.

The fibro-osseous tunnel has two bony (hamate and pisiform) and two fibrous (piso-hamate ligament and the tendinous arch) walls. The piso-hamate ligament has been considered the most important in compression.[80] The tendinous arch connects the pisiform and the hook of the hamate bone and serves as the origin of the adductor digiti minimi, the flexor digiti minimi brevis, and the opponens digiti minimi, that is, some of the hypothenar muscles.

Only the palmaris brevis muscle, which gets its innervation from the superficial branch of the ulnar nerve, and the two ulnar lumbricals, the adductor pollicis, and the deep head of the flexor pollicis brevis muscles, which receive their supply from the deep branch of the ulnar nerve, are spared in this syndrome. Sparing of the abductor digiti minimi muscle that receives its motor branch proximal to the tunnel differentiates this syndrome from the ulnar tunnel syndrome of Guyon.

The mechanism of compression is trauma, including carpal bone fractures.

The symptoms of piso-hamate syndrome are all motor, as the deep branch has no sensory components. Since the palmaris brevis and abductor digiti quinti minimi continue to function, the motor impairment requires astute examination and conformation by EMG studies.

Treatment is usually conservative and consists of oral anti-inflammatory medications, short-term immobilization, and local corticosteroid injections. Surgical decompression usually requires release of the hypothenar muscles from their origin.

Cubital Tunnel Syndrome

Compression of the ulnar nerve at the elbow, commonly called the cubital tunnel syndrome, is a common nerve entrapment of the upper extremity, second only to the carpal tunnel syndrome in frequency.

This syndrome, recognized for over 100 years,[81] is apparently becoming increasingly common due to the increasing use of computers, which involves repetitive use of the upper extremity held in an elbow flexed position and places direct pressure upon the nerve at the cubital tunnel (Fig. 2–63). The ulnar nerve is very superficial at this site.

At the elbow, the ulnar nerve enters the cubital groove on the posterior aspect of the medial epicondyle, where the roof of the tunnel is formed by an aponeurotic band at a transverse angle to the nerve. As the nerve leaves the tunnel it passes between the two heads of the flexor carpi ulnaris muscle.

The aponeurotic band stabilizes the ulnar nerve behind the medial epicondyle and prevents subluxation of the nerve during elbow actions. Hypermobility of the nerve exists,[82] however, and makes compression

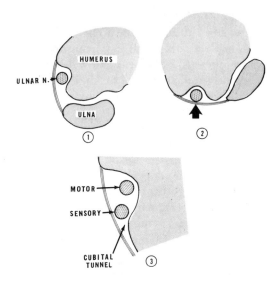

Figure 2–63. Cubital tunnel —ulnar nerve. In the supinated elbow (1) the ulnar nerve is removed from possible compression, whereas pronation (2) encourages pressure. The sensory component is depicted as compared with the motor fibers (3).

"outside" the canal possible. The retinaculum is lax in elbow extension and taut only in full flexion.[83] With flexion, the volume of the cubital tunnel decreases so that there is more pressure upon the nerve.[84] The cubital pressure also is found to be increased with the wrist extended and the shoulder forward flexed and abducted, a posture used in many occupations.[85]

Within the tunnel the motor fibers supplying the intrinsics of the hand are superficial, and those supplying the flexor carpi ulnaris and the digitorum profundus are deeper.[86] The superficial location of the sensory nerves (see Fig. 2–58) also explains the impaired sensation seen early in this syndrome.

More proximal to the cubital tunnel, the ulnar nerve passes under the "arcade of Struthers," which is a thick fascial band running from the medial head of the triceps muscle to the medial intermuscular septum.[87] This may also be a site of entrapment.

As symptoms from entrapment at the site are often delayed the term "tardy ulnar palsy" has evolved.[88] Surgical findings in this syndrome revealed a "markedly swollen and adherent ulnar nerve within the groove, with no significant elbow deformity." All patients operated on for release of the arch "without nerve transposition" had relief of symptoms.[89]

Symptoms of Cubital Tunnel Ulnar Nerve Compression. Aching pain on the medial site of the elbow near the medial epiconyle is frequently associated with "shooting" pains in the ulnar aspect of the hand and little finger. This hypesthesia is activity-related—provoked by elbow flexion and occasionally relieved by elbow extension. Unlike the carpal tunnel syndrome, the paresthesias are not nocturnal. Clumsiness of hand activities may be a complaint, depending upon the degree of motor involvement.

A positive Tinel sign may be elicited, but care must be exercised in eliciting this sign, since normal ulnar nerves at the elbow respond to excessive tapping. The sensory modality tests previously described (light touch, vibration, Semmes-Weinstein monofilament, and two-point discrimination) are diagnostic of nerve involvement.

A provocative test is flexing the elbow fully and extending the wrist for 3 minutes.[90] Motor evaluation begins with weakness of the first dorsal interosseus (resisting index finger abduction) and abductor digiti minimi (testing little finger abduction). Ultimately the presence of atrophy in the hypothenar region and the first web, with clawing of the ring and little finger, becomes apparent. A positive Froment sign (pinching a piece of paper between thumb and side of the index finger) is apparent. In this sign the distal thumb joint is flexed.

The major nerves to test are the flexor carpi ulnaris (testing wrist flexion in an ulnar direction) and the ulnar portion of the flexor digitorum profundus (testing flexion of the distal interphalangeal joint).[91] The normalcy of the bony aspect of the tunnel can be evaluated radiologically with special views.[92]

Treatment. Prevention is obviously desirable, that is avoidance of direct pressure upon the flexed elbow. If possible, moderate flexion with cushioning is desirable. Compression induced by sleep position must be identified and modified, for example, by using a small pillow to maintain elbow extension and avoid flexion. Modification of vocational activities must also be addressed. Frequent and forceful elbow flexion may also be incriminated and, when identified, must be eliminated.

Oral anti-inflammatory nonsteroidal medication has value, and perineural steroid injection has been proposed.[93] The disadvantage with the latter is subcutaneous atrophy and cosmetic skin depigmentation. In attempting tunnel injection the patient must be warned of these possibilities.

Surgical Intervention. There exists a controversy over which surgical approach affords the greatest benefit. The degree of preoperative compression strongly influences the chance of success, with those cases exhibiting intrinsic muscle weakness and atrophy having the poorest prognosis.[94]

Procedures vary from simple decompression to anterior transposition and medial epicondylectomy. The procedures are beyond the scope of this text, and the choice of procedure resides in the realm of the expert surgeon.

REFERENCES

1. Kalaska JF, Crammond DJ: Cerebral cortical mechanisms of reaching movements. Science 255:1517–1523, 1992.
2. Schmidt RF: Fundamentals of Neurophysiology. Springer-Verlag, New York, 1978.
3. Kandel ER, Hawkins RD: The biological basis of learning and individuality. Sci Am 79–86, 1992.
4. Barinaga M: Research news: the brain remaps its own contour. Science 9:216–218, 1992.
5. Talbot JD, Marrett S, Evans AC, Meyer E, Bushnell MC, Duncan GH: Multiple representations of pain in the human cerebral cortex. Science 251:1355–1358, 1991.
6. Melzack R: Central pain syndromes and theories of pain. In Casey KL (ed): Pain and Central Nervous System Disease. The Central Pain Syndrome. Raven Press, New York, 1991, pp 59–64.
7. Sunderland S: Nerve and Nerve Injuries. Livingstone, Edinburgh, 1968.
8. Sedden HJ: Three types of nerve injury. Brain 66:237–288, 1943.
9. Denny-Brown D, Brenner C: Lesion in peripheral nerve resulting from compression by spring clip. Arch Neurol Psychiatr 52:1–19, 1944.
10. Lundborg G: Nerve regeneration and repair: A review. Acta Orthop Scand 58:145–169, 1987.
11. Gundersen RW: Sensory neurite growth cone guidance by substrate absorbed nerve growth factor. J Neurosci Res 13:199–212, 1985.
12. Cailliet R: Pain mediated though the sympathetic nervous system. In Cailliet R: Pain: Mechanisms and Management, Philadelphia, FA Davis, 1993, pp 29–53.
13. Martin JH: Receptor physiology and submodality coding in the somatic sensory system. In Kandel ER and Swartz JH (eds): Principles of Neural Science, ed 2. Elsevier, New York, 1985, pp 287–300.
14. Louis et al.: Evaluation of normal values for stationary and moving two point discrimination in the hand. Hand Surg 9A:552, 1984.
15. Bell JA: Light touch-deep pressure testing using Semmes-Weinstein monofilaments. In Hunter, et al. (eds): Rehabilitation of the Hand. CV Mosby, Philadelphia, 1990, pp 585–593.
16. Sunderland S: Nerves and Injuries, ed 2. Churchill Livingstone, New York, 1978.
17. Kimura J: Electrodiagnosis in Diseases of Nerve and Muscle: Principles and Practice. FA Davis, Philadelphia, 1989, p 64.
18. Beasley R: Hand Injuries. WB Saunders, Philadelphia, 1981, p 278.
19. Holmes W, Young JZ: Nerve regeneration after immediate and delayed suture. J Anat 77:63, 1942.
20. Ramon-Y-Cajal S: Degeneration and Regeneration of the Nervous System, Vol 1. Oxford University Press, London, 1928.
21. Spencer PS: Morphology of the injured peripheral nerve. In Daniel RK, Terzis JK (eds): Reconstructive Microsurgery. Little, Brown, Boston, 1977, p 342.
22. Sunderland S: Nerve and Nerve Injuries. E & S Livingstone, Edinburgh, 1968.
23. Skirven T: Nerve injuries. In Stanley BG, Tibuzi M (eds): Concepts in Hand Rehabilitation, CPR. FA Davis, Philadelphia, 1992, pp 322–352.
24. Smith KL: Wound healing. In Stanley BG, Tibuzi SM (eds): Concepts of Hand Rehabilitation, CPR. FA Davis, Philadelphia, 1992, pp 35–56.
25. Madden JW, Peacock EE: Studies on the biology of collagen during wound healing. III: dynamic metabolism of scar collagen and remodeling of dermal wounds. Ann Surg 174:511, 1971.
26. Michlovitz S, Segal LR: Physical agents and electrotherapy techniques in hand reha-

bilitation. In Stanley BG, Tribuzi SM (eds): Concepts in Hand Rehabilitation, CPR. FA Davis, Philadelphia, 1992, pp 216–237.

27. McMiken D, Todd-Smith M, Thompson C: Strengthening of human quadriceps muscle by cutaneous electrical stimulation. Scand J Rehabil Med, 15:25, 1983.

28. Kramer J, Semple J: Comparison of selected strengthening techniques for normal quadriceps. Physiotherapy Canada 35:300, 1983.

29. Herbison GJ, Teng C, Gordon EE: Electrical stimulation of re-inervating rat muscle. Arch Phys Med Rehabil 54:156, 1973.

30. Rudge P: Tourniquet paralysis with prolonged conduction block: an electrophysiological study. J Bone Joint Surg (Br) 56:716–720, 1974.

31. Lundborg G: Ischemia nerve injury. Scand J Plast Reconstr Surg Hand Surg (Suppl) 6:1–113, 1970.

32. Ochoa J, Fowler TJ, Gilliatt RW: Anatomical changes in peripheral nerves compressed by a pneumatic tourniquet. J Anat 113:433–455, 1972.

33. Szabo RM, Chidgey LK: Stress carpal tunnel pressures in patients with carpal tunnel syndrome and normal patients. J Hand Surg (Am) 14:624–627, 1989.

34. Szabo RM, Madison M: Carpal tunnel syndrome. In: Common Hand Problems, Orthop Clin North Am, 23:103–109, 1992.

35. Phalen GS: The carpal tunnel syndrome. J Bone Joint Surg (Am) 48A:211, 1966.

36. Spinner RJ, Bachman JW, Amadio PC: The many faces of carpal tunnel syndrome. Mayo Clin Proc 64:829, 1989.

37. Braun RM, Davidson K, Doehr S: Provocative testing in the diagnosis of dynamic carpal tunnel syndrome. J Hand Surg 14A:195, 1989.

38. Luchetti R, Schoenhuber R, Alfarano M, et al.: Carpal tunnel syndrome: correlation between pressure measurement and intraoperative electrophysiological nerve study. Muscle Nerve 13:1164, 1990.

39. Szabo RM, Gelberman RH: Peripheral nerve compression: etiology, critical pressure threshold, and clinical assessment. Orthopedics 7:146, 1984.

40. Kuschner SH, Ebramzadeh E, Johnson D, Brien WW, Sherman R: Tinel's sign and Phalen's test in carpal tunnel syndrome (original research). Orthopedics 15:1297–1302, 1992.

41. Tinel J: Le signe du "formillement" dans les lesions des nerfs peripherique. Presse Med 47:388–389, 1915.

42. Brain WR, Wright AD, Wilkinson M: Spontaneous compression of both median nerves in the carpal tunnel. Six cases treated surgically. Lancet 1:277–282, 1947.

43. Phalen GS, Gardner WJ, LaLonde AA: Neuropathy of the median nerve due to compression beneath the transverse carpal ligament. J Bone Joint Surg 32A:109–112, 1950.

44. Phalen GS, Kendrick JJ: Compression neuropathy of the median nerve in the carpal tunnel. JAMA 164:524–530, 1947.

45. Phalen GS: The carpal tunnel syndrome. Clinical evaluation of 598 hands. Clin Orthop 83:29–40, 1972.

46. Goodman HV, Foster JB: Effect of local corticosteroid injection on median nerve conduction in carpal tunnel syndrome. Ann Phys Med 6:287, 1962.

47. Davlin LB, Aulicino PL, Bergfield TL: Anatomical variations of the median nerve at the wrist. A review paper. Orthop Rev 955–959, 1992.

48. Lanz U: Anatomical variations of the median nerve in the carpal tunnel. J Hand Surg (Am) 2:44–53, 1977.

49. Chow JC: Endoscopic release of the carpal ligament: a new technique for carpal tunnel syndrome. Arthroscopy 5:19–24, 1989.

50. Resnick CT, Miller BW: Endoscopic carpal tunnel release using the subligamentous two-portal technique. Contemp Orthop 22:269–277, 1991.

51. Clayton ML, Linscheid RL: Carpal tunnel surgery. Should the incision be above or below the wrist? Orthopaedics 11:819, 1988.
52. Curtis RM, Eversman WW Jr: Internal neurolysis as an adjunct to the treatment of the carpal tunnel syndrome. J Bone Joint Surg (Am) 55A:733, 1973.
53. Okutsu I, Ninomiya S, Takatori Y, Hamanaka I, Genba K, Ugawa Y, Schonholtz GJ, Okumura Y: Results of endoscopic management of carpal tunnel syndrome. Orthop Rev 81–87, 1993.
54. Gartsman GM, Kovach JC, Crouch CC, et al.: Carpal arch alteration after carpal tunnel syndrome release. J Hand Surg (Am) 11A:372, 1986.
55. Newmeyer WL: Editorial thoughts on the technique of carpal tunnel release. J Hand Surg (Am) 17A:985–986, 1992.
56. Chow JCY: Endoscopic release of the carpal ligament for carpal tunnel syndrome: 22-month clinical results. Arthroscopy 6:288–296, 1990.
57. Parenmark G, Alfram A-A, Malmkvist A-K: The significance of work tasks for rehabilitation outcome after carpal tunnel surgery. J Occup Rehabil 2:89–94, 1992.
58. Silverstein BA, Fine LJ, Armstrong TJ: Occupational factors and carpal tunnel syndrome. Am J Ind Med 11:343–358, 1987.
59. Hybbinette C-H, Mannerfelt L: The carpal tunnel syndrome. A retrospective study of 400 operated patients. Acta Orthop Scan 46:610–620, 1975.
60. Thorngren K-G, Werner CO: Normal grip strength. Acta Orthop Scand 50:255–259, 1979.
61. Gellman H, Kan D Gee V, Kuschber SH, Botte MJ: Analysis of pinch and grip strength after carpal tunnel release. J Hand Surg (Am) 14(A):863–865, 1989.
62. Hagberg M, Wegman DH: Prevalence rates and odds ratios of shoulder-neck diseases in different occupational groups. Br J Ind Med 44:602–610, 1987.
63. Fisset J, Roucq D, LaHaye T: Effets de la reconstruction du care dans la chirurgie du syndrome du canal carpient. Acta Orthop Belg 47:375, 1981.
64. Ilic A, Lolic V, Dimcevic S: Acta Orthop Lugosl 3:193, 1971.
65. Kopell HP, Thompson WA: Peripheral Entrapment Neuropathies. Williams & Wilkins, Baltimore, 1963.
66. Pecina MM, Krmpotic-Nemanic J, Markiewitz AD: Tunnel Syndromes. CRC Press, Boca Raton, Fla., 1991, pp 31–34.
67. Morris MH, Peters BH: J Neurol Neurosurg Psychiatry 39:461, 1976.
68. Spinner M: Injuries to the Major Branches of Peripheral Nerves of the Forearm, ed 2, WB Saunders, Philadelphia, 1978.
69. Commandre F: Pathologie abarticulaire. Lab Certane, Paris, 1977.
70. Hartz CR, Linscheid RL, Gramse RR, Daube JR: J Bone Joint Surg (Am) 63A:885, 1981.
71. Guyon F: Bull Soc Anat (Paris) 6:184, 1861.
72. Shea JD, McClain EJ: J Bone Joint Surg (Am) 51A:1095, 1969.
73. Davlin LB, Bergfield TG, Aulicino PL: Variations of the ulnar nerve: a surgical perspective. Orthop Rev 33–39, 1993.
74. Pecina M, Grospie R: Riv Pathol Aparato Locom 1:183, 1981.
75. Payan J: Electrophysiological localization of ulnar nerve lesions. J Neurol Neurosurg Psychiatry 32:208, 1969.
76. Hart VL, Gaynov V: J Bone Joint Surg 23:382, 1941.
77. Kleimert HE, Hayes JE: Plast Reconstr Surg 47:21, 1971.
78. Wissinger HA: Plast Reconstr Surg 56:501, 1975.
79. Uriburu TJF, Morchio FJ, Marin JC: J Bone Joint Surg (Am) 58A:145, 1976.
80. Hayes JR, Mulholland RC, O'Connor BT: J Bone Joint Surg (Am) 51A:1095, 1969.
81. MacKinnon SE, Dellon AL: Ulnar nerve entrapment at the elbow. In Surgery of the Peripheral Nerve. New York, Thieme Medical Publishers, 1988, pp 217.

82. Childress HM: Recurrent ulnar nerve dislocation at the elbow. J Bone Joint Surg (Am) 38A:978, 1956.
83. O'Driscoll SW, Horii E, Carmichael SW, et al.: The anatomy of the cubital tunnel and its relationship to ulnar neuropathies (abstract SS-03) In: Abstracts of the American Society for Surgery of the Hand 45th Annual Meeting, Toronto, 1990, pp 3–11.
84. Kumar K, Deshpande S, Jain M, et al.: Evaluation of various fibro-osseous tunnel pressures (carpal, cubital and tarsal) in normal human subjects. Ind J Physiol Pharmacol 32:139, 1988.
85. Macnicol MF: Extraneural pressures affecting the ulnar nerve at the elbow. Hand 14:5, 1982.
86. Sunderland S: The intraneural topography of the radial, median and ulnar nerves. Brain 68:243, 1945.
87. Kane E, Kaplan EBN, Spinner M: Observations of the course of the ulnar nerve in the arm. Ann Chir 27:487, 1973.
88. Feindel W, Stratford J: The role of the cubital tunnel in tardy ulnar palsy. Can J Surg 1:287, 1958.
89. Buerhler MJ, Thayer DT: The elbow flexion test. A clinical test for the cubital tunnel syndrome. Clin Orthop 233:213, 1988.
90. Vanderpool DW: Peripheral compression lesions of the ulnar nerve. J Bone Joint Surg (Br) 50B:792, 1968.
91. St. John JN, Palmaz JC: The cubital tunnel in ulnar entrapment neuropathy. Radiology 158:119, 1986.
92. Pechan J, Kredba J: Treatment of cubital tunnel syndrome by means of local administration of cortisonoids. Acta Univ Carol (Med) (Praha) 26:125, 1980.
93. Foster RJ, Edshage S: Factors related to the outcome of surgically managed compressive ulnar neuropathy at the elbow level. J Hand Surg (Am) 6:181, 1981.
94. McPherson SA, Meals RA: Cubital tunnel syndrome. In Common hand problems, Szabo RM (ed) Orthop Clin North Am 23:111–123, 1992.

CHAPTER 3
Reflex Sympathetic Dystrophy

There are many neurological disorders that affect the upper extremities. These include compartment syndromes;[1] referred neurological diseases, for example, cervical radiculitis; and upper motor neuron disorders, for example, stroke; however, the most challenging of pain disorders are the sympathetic afflictions that have become termed reflex sympathetic dystrophy (RSD).

HISTORICAL BACKGROUND

Burning pain of an extremity following injury was noted by Paré in the 16th century,[2] but it received more consideration during the Civil War, when it was described in wounded soldiers who sustained peripheral nerve injuries.[3] Mitchell, who described this injury sequel, employed the term "causalgia," as the patients all complained of "burning pain." Letievant, in 1873, discussed causalgia and related disorders with vivid descriptions.[5]

Leriche associated the sympathetic nervous system with the genesis of this syndrome and he claimed that this relationship was the reason for his success in treating the condition by periarterial sympathectomy and later by blocking the sympathetic chain with procaine.[6] Electrical stimulation of the sympathetic efferents in patients with causalgia has been reported to cause pain,[7] which again implicates the sympathetic nervous system.

The syndrome was associated with trauma and was characterized by various degrees of burning, aching pain, vasomotor and other autonomic disturbances, and gradual progressive dystrophic tissue changes. Bonica considered causalgia as a "major" syndrome under the broad generic

132

term of reflex sympathetic dystrophy (RSD).[6] Involvement of the hand and fingers is also noted in "minor" categories of RSD, in which pain, burning or otherwise, is of lesser significance and may be absent.

The lack of homogeneity in the classification of RSD syndromes as to mechanisms, pathogenesis, and response to therapy[9] lead to the issuing of a definition by a taxonomy subcommittee of the International Association for the Study of Pain (IASP).[10] In this definition, causalgia was described as "a syndrome of sustained burning pain after traumatic nerve lesion combined with vasomotor and sudomotor dysfunction and later trophic changes." As with Bonica's classification, "causalgia" remains a major category under reflex sympathetic dystrophy (RSD).

The Sixth World Congress on Pain held in Adelaide offered an operational definition:

> "RSD is a descriptive term meaning a complex disorder or group of disorders that may develop as a consequence of trauma affecting the limbs, with or without obvious nerve lesion. RSD may also develop after visceral diseases, and central nervous system lesions or, rarely, without an obvious antecedent event. It consists of pain and related sensory abnormalities in the motor system and changes in the structure of both superficial and deep tissues ("trophic" changes). It is not necessary that all components are present. It is agreed that the name "reflex sympathetic dystrophy" is used in a descriptive sense and does not imply specific underlying mechanisms.

The last statement emphasizes that the definition avoids indicating mechanisms. It is also apparent that "pain" need not be a significant or major component, but is rarely absent.

Associated with causalgic pain, hyperalgesia and allodynia (pain caused by non-noxious stimuli) are also noted in the affected area. A combination of causalgia, hyperalgesia, and allodynia becomes a homogeneous syndrome, whether or not there is, or was, a nerve lesion, and the underlying pathophysiologic mechanism is the same as in RSD.[11]

The resultant dystrophy involves wasting of tissues such as muscle and bone, and abnormal growth features such as ridging of the nails and hyperkeratosis of the skin. The dystrophic changes are secondary to vasomotor imbalance, whereas the local vasochemical changes are caused by initial trauma (Fig. 3–1).

MECHANISMS AND PATHOGENESIS

Over the centuries there have evolved numerous theories regarding the pathogenesis of sympathetic mediated pain. These theories may be variously described as "peripheral" or "central."

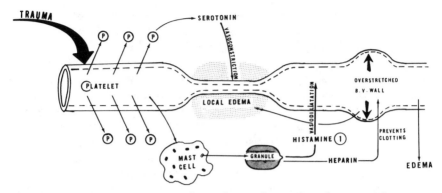

Figure 3–1. Schematic concept of vasochemical sequelae of trauma. The micro-hemorrhage or macrohemorrhage releases serotonin which causes vasoconstriction and releases mast cells. The granules of these mast cells release histamine, which causes vasodilation with resultant edema.

Peripheral Hypothesis

It has been proposed that algesic substances are liberated at the periphery and that these initiate local hyperesthesia and the pain transmission sequence (Fig. 3–2).[12] These latter involve the formation of synapses within the transmission system at the dorsal root ganglion and the dorsal horn (Fig. 3–3). Loss of inhibition due to damage of the large myelinated fibers has also been postulated.[13]

Except in the endings of sensory nerve afferents, the midsection of a normal nerve is incapable of generating impulses. Damaged nerves undergo changes that transform them from impulse conductors to impulse "generators" from depolarization-forming ectopic pacemakers.[14] The resultant "efferent" activity releases catecholamines, including noradrenaline. When these bind with α-adrenergic receptors, the receptors give off repetitive discharges, thus becoming "generators" (Fig. 3–4). The formation of sympathetic terminal receptors containing α-adrenergic substances has recently been advanced[14] (see Fig. 3–5) to support the regenerating afferent fiber neuroma concept of Wall and Gutnick[15] (Fig. 3–6).

Central Hypothesis

Increased peripheral activity allegedly induces more central hyperactivity and hypersensitivity, beginning at the dorsal horn of the cord in Rexed layers I–II (Fig. 3–7), as well as convergence of the afferent nociceptor and mechanoreceptor activity at the wide-dynamic-range

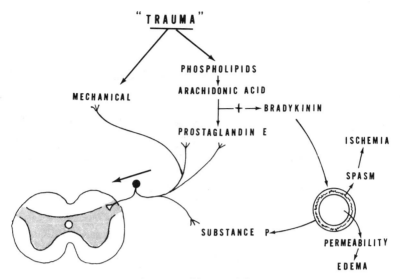

Figure 3-2. Nociceptive substances liberated from trauma. Regardless of the type of trauma the traumatized tissue liberates breakdown products from phospholipids into arachodinic acid and ultimately prostaglandins. The trauma also affects the blood vessels, causing spasm, edema and liberation of platelets that break down to liberate serotonin and substance P. Other kinins and toxic substances are nociceptive products that irritate nerve endings, ultimately causing pain.

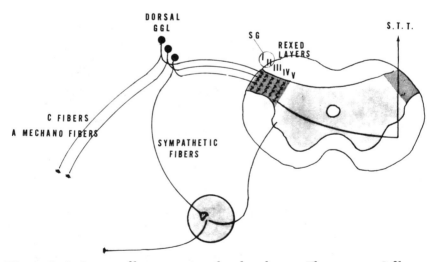

Figure 3-3. Sensory fibers entering the dorsal root. The sensory C-fibers, mechano A fibers, and sympathetic sensory afferent fibers enter the dorsal horn into the dorsal horn of the cord grey matter. The dorsal horn is divided into numerous (I–V or more layer of Rexed) where the main sensory fibers enter Rexed I and II, which constitute the substantia gelatinosum (SG). Sensory impulses traverse the cord to ascend in the spinothalamic tracts (S.T.T.). One third of unmyelinated C-fibers are considered to enter the dorsal column via the motor roots of the anterior horn (not shown in illustration).

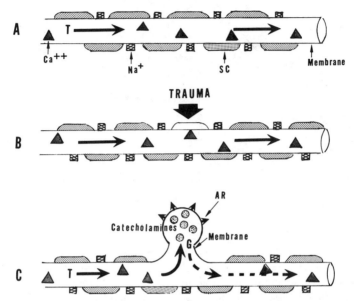

Figure 3-4. Ectopic generator evolving from nerve injury. (A) Normal nerve, which is a transmitter (T) of impulses within the membrane. The Schwann cells (SC) of the membrane form the myelin sheath. The electrolytes sodium (Na$^+$) and calcium (Ca^{++}) generate the impulse. (B) Trauma damages the Schwann cells of the membrane. (C) At the site of trauma there is a release of catecholamines and the membrane forms a saccule containing these catecholamines which become generators (G) of abnormal impulses (broken line). Adrenergic receptors (AR) form on the membrane surface of the saccule explaining the hypersensitivity of the nerve at that site. (Modified from Devor M: Nerve pathophysiology and mechanisms of pain in causalgia. J Autonomic Nervous System 7:371–384, 1983, Elsevier Biomedical Press.)

(WDR) cells in laminae IV–VI.[16] Repeated electrical stimulation of unmyelinated nerve fibers has been shown to enlarge the receptive fields in the spinal horn neurons.[17-19]

This plasticity (enlargement) of the WDR cells can explain superficial hypersensitivity, in that the same peripheral stimulus excites a larger sensory field in the dorsal horn.[20] Regions previously responsive only to intense stimuli now respond to usually innocuous mechanical stimuli.[21] This plasticity of the receptive area was confirmed in the trigeminal receptive area in the nucleus proprius,[22] an area which is similar to the dorsal horn of the cord.

Melzack[23] considered causalgic pain to result from the loss of normal sensory input (Fig. 3–8) ascending to the brainstem reticular system from the periphery (Fig. 3–9). This sensory input normally exerts a tonic inhibitory influence upon the ascending nociceptive system.

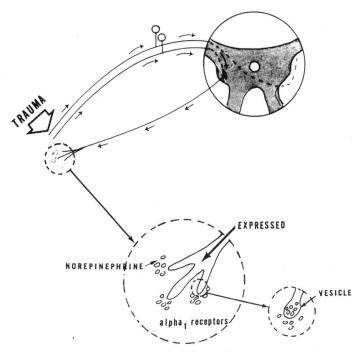

Figure 3–5. Nociceptor activation of alpha-1 adrenoreceptors. Trauma causes the sympathetic nerves going to the area to "express" norepinephrine that is contained within the vesicles. The liberated norepinephrine reacts with the α_1-receptors to cause causalgic symptoms.

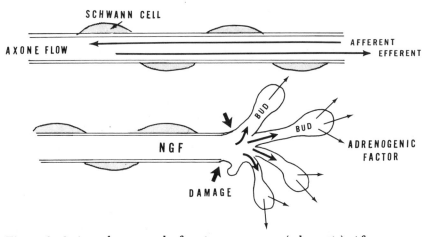

Figure 3–6. Axonal outgrowths forming a neuroma (schematic). After a nerve injury with compression or partial to total severance, the nerve growth factor (NGF) stimulates the nerve to advance distally and form "buds," which create more endings than the normal nerve shown in the upper drawing. By virtue of the greater secretion of adrenogenic factors, the nerve becomes more sensitive to adrenogenic agonists and transmits more potential pain fiber impulses to the spinal cord (see also Fig. 3–10).

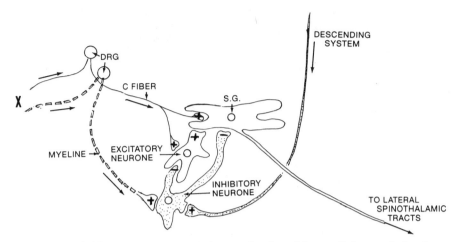

Figure 3–7. Nociceptive transmission to the dorsal horn of the cord. A schematic version of nociceptive transmission to the dorsal horn is presented. X is the noxious stimulus that is transmitted through afferent C-fibers and myelinated large diameter fibers. In the substantia gelatinosum (S.G.) of the dorsal horn the impulses go to and activate (+) the transmission cell of the S.G. Impulses from the myelinated fibers activate the inhibitory neurones (−), which modulate the projection cell. Ultimately the impulses are transmitted to the lateral spinothalamic tracts where they ascend to the thalamus. The descending tracts also modulate the impulses arriving at the transmission cells.

Carron considers RSD to be similar to the denervation hyperesthesia noted after surgical interruption of the sympathetic nervous system.[24] This occurs in three stages:

1. The denervation phase with an increased blood flow.
2. The hypersensitivity phase resulting from the circulating catecholamines.
3. The reinnervation phase characterized by excessive adrenergic growth.

Roberts proposed a causative hypothesis for RSD and causalgia based on two assumptions:[25] first, there is a high rate of firing of the wide-dynamic-range neurons, second, these neurons become activated by non-nociceptive impulses (Fig. 3–10). These processes occur at the dorsal horn level, but are now also known to occur at the dorsal root level and at more central levels in the midbrain area.

This hypothesis explains the hypersensitivity of extremities afflicted with RSD.

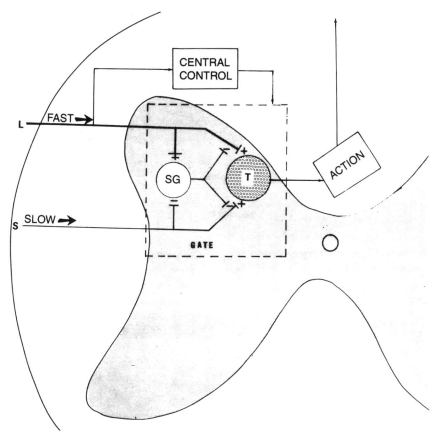

Figure 3–8. "Gate" theory of Wall and Melzack. The gray area is the dorsal horn of the cord. The Rexed layers I and II are the substantia gelatinosum (SG). The sensory afferent fibers carrying nociception are the "slow" C fiber neurons that activate (+) the SG. The impulses then proceed via the fibers ascending to the reticular formation via spinoreticulothalamic tracts and the spinothalamic tracts (STTs) to the thalamus and the reticular system. These impulses are ultimately interpreted at the cortex as pain. Fast fibers (A-α) and mechano (A-Δ) (I) fibers are inhibitory (−) in that they modulate the intensity of the slower fiber activity.

Natural Opioid Modulation. "Failed" natural opioid modulation in regional sympathetic ganglia has been considered as a possible cause of RSD.[26] After injury to a limb, there is normally a rise in opioid modulation within a dorsal root ganglion in that region, to avoid excessive autonomic activity (Fig. 3–11). After a trivial injury in a susceptible individual, this increased modulation may fail or be inadequate.

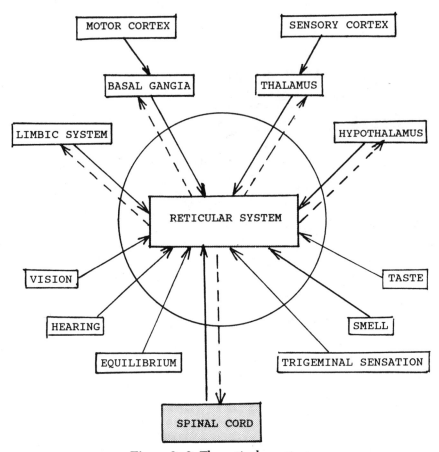

Figure 3–9. The reticular system.

After injury, opioid "withdrawal" is exhibited in the presence of RSD. Among these withdrawal signs and symptoms are altered cutaneous sensation, increased pilomotor activity, excessive sweating and vascular instability causing skin color changes, swelling, and warmth. If opioid modulation fails after injury to a limb, all the above signs and symptoms (of RSD) can occur.

Regional Nerve Blocks. The presence of opioid peptides and their receptors in sympathetic ganglia[27,28] and consideration of "withdrawal" signs have prompted injection of morphine or a similar derivative into the stellate root ganglion in RSD patients who have not received benefit from anesthetic agent stellate blocks.

In patients with RSD that is being treated by morphine injection into the stellate ganglion, no significant autonomic changes occur, but pain is relieved, and the tonic muscle spasm typically found in RSD

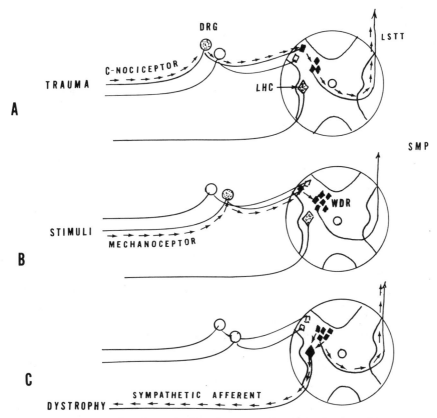

Figure 3-10. Postulated neurophysiologic mechanism of sympathetic maintained pain (SMP). The transmission via C-nociceptor fibers (A) of impulses from the peripheral tissues that have been traumatized and created peripheral nociceptor chemicals (see details in text). These impulses pass through the dorsal root ganglion (DRG) to activate the grey matter of the cord in the Rexed layers. When sensitized, they are termed *wide dynamic range neurones* (WDR). The WDR, becoming very irritated, receives impulses from the periphery via the A-mechanoreceptors fibers, (B) which normally transmit sensations of touch, vibration, temperature, etc. When the periphery is stimulated, (skin touch, pressure, or joint movement) these impulses enhance and maintain the irritability of the WDR. The impulses from the WDR continue cephalad through the lateral spinal thalamic tracts (LSTT) to the thalamic centers with resultant continued pain. The WDR impulses irritate the lateral horn cells (LHC), which generate sympathetic impulses that innervate the peripheral tissues resulting in the symptoms and findings of dystrophy (C).

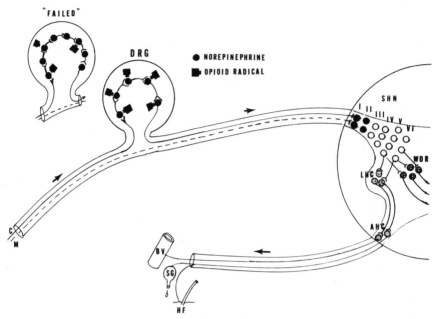

Figure 3-11. Opioid modulation of pain in the dorsal root ganglion after trauma: "failed modulation." There are opioid radicals in the normal dorsal root ganglia (DRG) that modulate the norepinephrine contained within the small saccules in the ganglion. Normally afferent impulses from C fibers (C) transmitting nociceptive impulse to the spinal horn nuclei (SHN) impinge upon Rexed layers I-II. These impulses react with wide-dynamic range cells (WDR) in the cord (Rexed layer VII) with impulses going cephalad to the lateral spinothalamic tract (small arrows). Fibers connect the Rexed layers cells with lateral horn cells (LHC) that innervate the sympathetic fibers to blood vessels (BV), sweat glands (SG) and hair follicles (HF). Repeated or intense nociceptive impulses increase ("plasticity") the number of norepinephrine cells within the dorsal root ganglia increasing sensitivity to even mechanoreceptor (M) impulses hence allodynia. In "failed" opioid modulation (*upper left drawing*) the epinephrine cells are increased and the opioid radicals proportionately decreased hence bombardment to SHN is increasing the number of WDR cells.

decreases. The restoration of muscle strength in the upper extremity is valuable in preventing the subsequent dystrophic changes attributed to disuse in this condition. That this is not a systemic benefit is seen from the fact that with systemic injection of opioids a similar release of muscle spasm does not occur.

It is of interest that RSD occurs relatively frequently from trivial injuries, which apparently fail to initiate or maintain sufficient opioid modulation. The frequent immobilization of a limb after injury may contribute to opioid modulation by interfering with the neural traffic invoked by activity. Effective therapy applied to RSD patients may actually restore opioid modulation and minimize or avoid dystrophic changes. Strenuous muscular exercises are known to increase blood concentrations of opioids.[29]

The Roberts theory of causalgia[25] may indicate how continued mechanoreceptor activity bombarding the wide-dynamic-range-neurons increases central hyperactivity. This is accompanied by an increased zone of sensitization in the dorsal horn. In the presence of sympathetic maintained pain, signs of sympathetic hyperactivity need not be present,[29] nor are they needed to diagnose RSD.

Trauma may or may not be ascertained to have occurred in RSD, or the trauma may be "trivial." Ascertaining a predisposition to RSD would be very desirable in order to initiate early or preventative treatment. Preexisting anxiety and/or stress, which increases the release of norepinephrine and thus increases arteriolar hyperactivity, may predispose to RSD.[30] This has misled many physicians to consider RSD as entirely "psychogenic," often to the detriment to the patient. A severe emotional stress often precedes the advent of RSD.[31] Smokers are known to be refractory to RSD treatment.[32]

Preoperative prophylactic opioid stellate ganglion block in hand surgery may prevent subsequent RSD, and it may allow the surgery to be performed without excessive bleeding, as is noted after a local anesthetic block.[33] When skin flap healing requires extra vascularity to the site, both injections can be used, as needed vascularity and avoidance of RSD is achieved.

Regional nerve blocks may decrease the sensitization of the wide-dynamic-range dorsal horn ganglia. (Sensitization is known to enhance the risk of RSD.) This consideration has increased the use of regional nerve blocks.[34] Hand surgery done under both the opioid stellate block and a local anesthetic block, even with general anesthesia, may prevent RSD.

Role of the Sympathetic Nervous System. Recently, numerous discussions by neuroscientists have questioned the precise role of the sympathetic nervous system in the causation of pain,[35] even though clinicians seem assured of its role. The value of sympathetic intervention and/or interruption is the basis for the controversy.

Decreased temperature of the symptomatic part may be due to increased sympathetic neural tone, which may not be the cause of pain. Hyperthermia may be due to antidromic nociceptor vasodilitation. A review of the original literature by S. Weir Mitchell,[36] led to rejection of the concept that causalgia was related to the sympathetic nervous system. W. K. Livingstone concluded that "one might start by abandoning, for the time being, the assumption that activities of the sympathetic nerves represent the essential factor in either the cause or the cure of the causalgia syndrome."[37]

J. Hannington-Kiff believes that "it is 'not' through sympathoparalysis that sympathetic blocks transiently relieve the condition."[38] The precise role of sympathetic blocks have not been confirmed by controlled studies with placebos.[39]

Regarding the role of the sympathetic nervous system in causing pain, a good experimental and clinical design model has yet to be created. The terms "reflex," "sympathetic," and "dystrophy" have gained an unscientific role in the postulated mechanism.[40]

That pain and the resultant dystrophic changes are caused by alterations in the peripheral blood flow as a result of sympathetic hyperactivity has not been substantiated by plethysmography, oscillometry, or fluorescein injection studies, although these have revealed "increases" in limb blood flow.

Roberts has suggested a model in which the mechanoreceptors stimulate the wide-dynamic-range neurons (WDR) and are responsible for allodynia (see Fig. 3–10).[41]

Other Considerations

The plea[35] by Ochoa is that "it is dangerous that the diagnosis of RSD is a potpourri label given without verification."[42]

The effect of psychological factors in contributing to the onset and persistence of the syndrome remain prominent in the medical literature[43] and justify these psychological factors being strongly considered in the management of RSD. Prevention of potential RSD in traumatized patients should be a paramount consideration in management, so as to minimize the necessity of treating the ultimate sequelae.[44]

DIAGNOSIS

Numerous diagnostic terms are currently applied to RSD syndromes including the following:

Algoneurodystrophy

Chronic traumatic edema

Minicausalgia

Minor causalgia

Peripheral trophoneurosis

Painful osteoporosis

Shoulder-hand-finger syndrome

Traumatic angiospasm

Sympathalgia

Post-traumatic pain syndrome

Reflex algodystrophy

Sudeck's atrophy

This plethora of terms further confuses the classification of various RSD syndromes. The diagnosis of a "major" reflex sympathetic dystrophy is suggested by history and physical findings.[45]

History:

- Pain out of proportion to the injury
- Pain described as "neuralgic" or "dysesthetic." Terms such as "burning," "numbness," "tingling," "itching" are often used.
- Pain that may be confined to a neurological dermatomal area but is more often diffuse, less precise, and of a vascular distribution
- Pain that is usually restricted to a distal peripheral limb although it may affect the face, tongue, or face
- Frequent absence of an objective neural lesion
- Accentuation of the pain by superficial non-noxious stimulus such as touch, air, or vibration
- Frequent occurrence of inappropriate behavioral responses such as seclusion and withdrawal

PHYSICAL FINDINGS

Patients who use terms to describe the pain that suggest a sympathetic component also seek help due to dystrophic changes. There are many cases that present with these dystrophic changes without causalgic pain.

There have been sequential "stages" of dystrophy described. Acute stages I and II and chronic stage III have been designated. Findings include the following:

- Soft puffy edema of the extremity
- Rubor or paleness (skin color changes)
- Cold or warm sensation of the skin
- Excessive moisture or dryness of the skin

- Increased hair or nail growth
- Edema progressing to induration
- Passive and active joint limitation
- Muscle atrophy
- Osteoporosis noted on x-ray studies of the involved extremity[47]
- Gradual atrophic arthritic changes of the joints of the involved extremity
- Pain relieved or diminished by a sympathetic intervention.[48] The controversy regarding the efficacy of this procedure has been discussed

A recent editorial comment in the journal *Pain* has classified reflex sympathetic dystrophy on the basis of history and physical findings of dystrophic changes as being a "full blown syndrome."[48]

There is confusion in arriving at a precise diagnosis of RSD in patients who have a causalgia type of pain of unknown etiology, and presenting only one or two of the dystrophic findings present in the "full-blown syndrome." The minimal features of the syndrome required to lead to a precise diagnosis of RSD remain unresolved. Janig addressed this quandary when he participated in an IASP committee developing a consensus definition of RSD.[49] The resultant decision specified that "RSD involved pain, not specifically 'burning' in quality, with 'abnormalities' of sensation, motor function, blood flow, with sweating and trophic changes in the skin and deep tissues of the involved extremity."

This vague definition did not specify the specific minimal "abnormalities" needed to make a precise diagnosis of RSD. Janig later proposed three types of RSD:[50]

1. Algodystrophy, which included pain and "all" features of dystrophy in what we have termed the "full-blown syndrome."
2. RSD without pain.
3. Sympathetically maintained pain (SMP).

Essentially his definition of RSD was pain accompanied by vasomotor sudomotor trophic changes that were unexplained by other causes.

"Relief by sympathetic nerve block" presented another conflict in the acceptance of these three classifications. Relief by local analgesic sympathetic block had been considered as necessary for a specific diagnosis of RSD.[51] This raised the question as to whether a diagnosis of RSD could be entertained if a sympathetic block was not effective. Another question raised was whether the anesthetic agent used in a sympathetic block affected the somatic nerves in the vicinity of the injection and/or whether the anesthetic agent (lidocaine) had a systemic absorption effect.

There are RSD-like syndromes, such as tissue damaged by nerve injury, that benefit from systemically administered lidocaine. There are also conditions of nerve damage that result in pain and allodynia, along with skin temperature changes and resultant atrophy, yet no involvement of the sympathetic system.[52,53] Lidocaine given intravenously has relieved neuropathic pains.[54]

The "specific" sensory abnormalities mentioned in the IASP definition include heat-induced hyperalgesia, low-threshold A-beta–mediated or high-threshold mechanical allodynia, and slow temporal summation of mechanical allodynia.[55] At present, the criteria for an accurate diagnosis of RSD remain to be clarified.

In the "minor" classification of Bonica[8] and Janig[51] falls the second type of RSD, that "without pain," here, the entity of shoulder-hand-finger syndrome (SHFS) frequently presents itself. There are numerous instances where this syndrome is found, such as:

- After a fracture
- After hemiparesis due to a vascular incident
- After myocardial infarction
- After compression, such as by an extremity cast
- After injection
- After shoulder peritendinitis, bursitis, fracture

This syndrome appears to be initiated by trauma, and frequently by minor trauma.

The sequelae of dystrophic changes appear to be vascular, as is evident in the "frozen" shoulder of the "full-blown" RSD (Fig. 3–12). A "full-blown RSD" can occur without pain in the shoulder-hand-finger syndrome.

CLINICAL MANIFESTATIONS OF RSD DYSTROPHY

The initial observable tissue reaction is dorsal edema of the fingers, with the skin appearing smooth, "puffy" and shiny. Dorsal edema is predominant, as there is a preponderance of veins and lymphatics in this dorsal region of the fingers. The wrinkles over the dorsum of the finger joints become obliterated. The edema may pit.

The fingers can no longer be fully flexed because the edematous fluid elevates the extensor tendons of the fingers (Fig. 3–13) and impairs the "pumping action" of the upper extremity. If the shoulder is also limited in range of motion, as frequently occurs in this syndrome, further "pumping action" is restricted (Fig. 3–14).

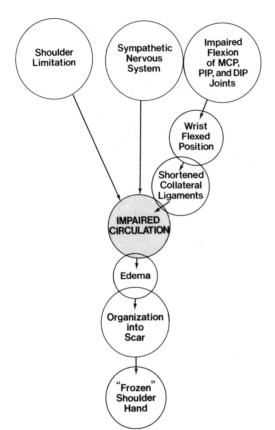

Figure 3–12. Sequences leading to "frozen" shoulder-hand-finger syndrome.

The edema seeps under the collateral ligaments of the digits making them "taut" in their extended position. Normally, due to the incongruity of these joints, the ligaments are slack in the extended position and become taut in full flexion (Fig. 3–15). The collateral ligaments, now taut because of the underlying edema, restrict flexion of the joint. Mechanical release of finger edema (Fig. 3–16) in conjunction with active and passive range of motion exercises has proven effective.

The untreated hand and fingers remain in a partially flexed position, and the periarticular tissues undergo contraction. The blood supply to the cartilage is impaired and gradually an atrophic arthritic condition occurs. The blood supply to bone is also restricted and results in osteoporosis. The skin undergoes ischemic atrophy and fibrous thickening, and the hair follicles hypertrophy. These tissue changes are the characteristic "full-blown" dystrophic hand changes seen in SHFS RSD.

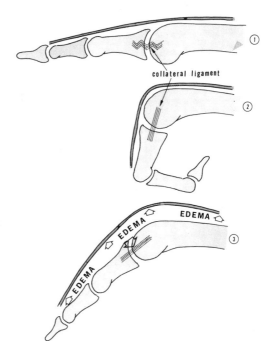

Figure 3–13. Finger changes in shoulder-hand-finger syndrome. (1) Normal extension of the metacarpophalangeal joint. Collateral ligaments are relaxed. (2) In normal flexion, the collateral ligaments become taut. (3) Edema occurs on the dorsum of the finger elevating the extensor tendons; this prevents flexion. The collateral ligaments become elevated in the extended finger position, causing them to be taut and preventing flexion.

TREATMENT OF THE REFLEX SYMPATHETIC DYSTROPHY SYNDROME

Assuming a correct diagnosis of RSD, "urgent" intervention is required to diminish the pain and intervene in the progression of the anticipated dystrophic changes, with often cause more impairment than pain alone.

On the basis of the pathomechanics of the syndrome the following treatment protocol is proposed:

- A meaningful explanation to the patient and family, in understandable terms, of the significance of the symptoms and findings
- Early active therapeutic involvement by a therapist, a family member, and the patient
- Local application of ice or heat depending on the vasodilatation (rubor, warm) or vasoconstriction (pale, cold) aspect of the overlying skin. In the presence of pain, ice is usually indicated and should be applied frequently and for sufficient periods of time
- Passive and active motion of "all" the joints of the extremity[56]

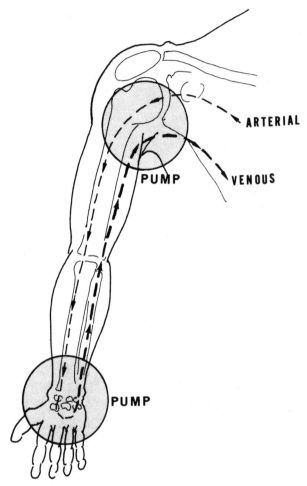

Figure 3–14. Venous lymphatic pumps of the upper extremity.

- Elevation of the involved extremity frequently and for prolonged periods of time. Dependent posture of the extremity must be avoided or minimized.
- Passive and active removal of the edema using compressive dressing or vasoconstrictive equipment[57]
- Injection of local "trigger areas with an anesthetic agent, with or without the addition of steroids
- Vasocoolant spray followed by stretch of the restricted myofascial tissues

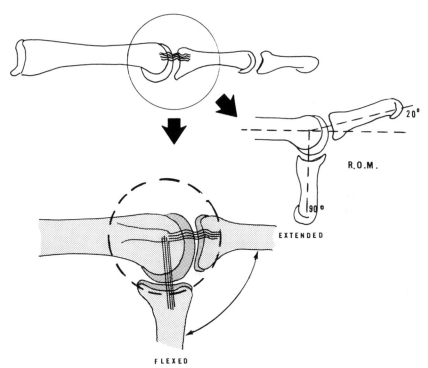

Figure 3–15. Metacarpophalangeal joints. As a result of the eccentric radius of rotation about the axis of the head of the metacarpal (*dotted circle*), flexion of the phalanx causes the collateral ligaments to become taut. The laxity of the ligaments in extension permits some lateral motion. Range of motion (ROM) is 90° flexion and 20° hyperextension.

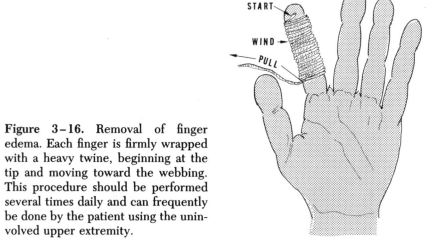

Figure 3–16. Removal of finger edema. Each finger is firmly wrapped with a heavy twine, beginning at the tip and moving toward the webbing. This procedure should be performed several times daily and can frequently be done by the patient using the uninvolved upper extremity.

- Local transcutaneous electric nerve stimulation (TENS) if pain is significant. This may be continued if application proves to be effective[58]
- Nerve block of the involved area with an anesthetic agent. This blocks the A-mechanoreceptors and the A-delta and C fibers, as well as sympathetic nerve fibers.
- Sympathetic nerve blocks (cervicothoracic or stellate ganglion nerve block). In refractory cases, a continuous sympathetic nerve blockade can be employed via an 18-gauge, 15-cm Teflon catheter inserted under roentgen vision to lie on the lateral portion of the anterior surface of the vertebral body of C7.[59] In the case of a refractory lower extremity RSD, lumbar sympathetic blocks can be administered every day for four sessions. If they are ineffectual, they should be discontinued; if they are effective, a surgical or chemical sympathectomy can be considered.[60] Cervical epidural injection of steroids has had recent advocacy.[61,62] Continuous epidural blockades have been effective in intractable pain.
- Stellate ganglion opioid (morphine) injection
- Bier blocks of the afflicted extremity.[63] With a tourniquet inflated to 100 mm above systolic blood pressure, a solution of guanethedine (10–40 mg), reserpine (1–2 mg), and 0.5% lidocaine is administered through a venous cannula. This block currently used in Europe, is not available in the United States. Parenteral reserpine is banned and parenteral guanethidine is still considered experimental.
- Sympathectomy. This is used when temporary chemical sympathetic blocks are effective but the symptoms return. It can be performed using 6% to 7% phenol or by radio frequency thermal application but surgical resection of the sympathetic nerves remains the standard approach.
- Nonsteroidal anti-inflammatory medication (NSAID). Considered early in the treatment this may have some value, but long-term results have been disappointing.
- Oral steroids (60–80 mg prednisone). A short (2 week) course followed by a 2-week tapering program has its advocates.
- Heterocyclic antidepressants.[64] Amitriptyline (10–50 mg HS) or trazadone (50–150 mg HS) have value.
- Carbamazepine (initial dose of 200 mg). Essentially an anticonvulsant, it has proven effective in trigeminal neuralgia[64] and has some benefit in RSD.
- Beta blockers (propranolol) and α-adrenergic blockers (prazosin[66] and phenoxybenzamine). All have been reported to be of value.
- Topical application of capsaicin.[67] This relieves the hypersensitivity of the affected region in many patients.

• Oral nifedipine, a calcium-channel blocker that induces peripheral vasodilitation. A dose of 10 mg three times daily for 1 week has proven effective. Increasing the dose to 30 mg three times a day for 3 weeks and then gradually decreasing the dose is effective if smaller doses have given some, but not sufficient, benefit.[68]

It is apparent from the proposed protocol that pain AND the dystrophic changes are all addressed. To address merely the pain and neglect the tissue changes leading to full-blown dystrophy leads to failure in treatment, as the dystrophic changes during their evolution cause pain, and ultimately lead to disability.

RELATED CONDITIONS

Vascular Impairment

Vascular impairment of the upper extremity can result from trauma, infection, or occlusive disease. The latter may evolve from embolic, thrombotic, neural, thermal, or mechanical pressure factors. Vascular impairment to tissues leads to scarring, muscle atrophy, joint contracture, or nerve entrapment.

Raynaud's Phenomenon

Etiology and Symptoms. This is a condition attributed to vasospasm triggered by exposure to external cold or emotional stress. It is most prevalent in women in their fourth decade and occurs bilaterally. An episode characteristically occurs with sudden pallor of the fingers approaching total blanching. As circulation returns there may be cyanosis followed by reflex vasodilitation (hyperemia).

Raynaud's phenomenon is a manifestation of vasomotor instability with abnormal sympathetic nervous system response to stress. There are numerous medical conditions that initiate this phenomenon, for example, "cervical thoracic outlet syndrome,"[69] or repetitive traumata, such as operating a pneumatic drill. Mechanical neurovascular compression of the brachial plexus and the subclavian arteries leads to the symptoms of Raynaud's phenomenon. Buerger's disease rarely affects the upper extremities.[70]

Raynaud's phenomenon may be the forerunner to scleroderma, which is a collagen vascular disease entity, but usually no disease can be associated with the phenomenon itself. That there is a relationship with the emotions[71] has been revealed by the techniques of biofeedback, employing digital temperature control during an examination.[72]

Exposure to extremes of external temperatures, especially in connection with moisture and wind, has been impuned. Chilblains are a mild reaction of the skin and result from exposure to temperatures ranging from freezing to 60°F. Here the skin assumes a red, swollen, warm appearance, with an itchy sensation.

Frostbite is essentially a first and second degree burn; the former causes redness (erythema) of the skin followed by desquamation, and the latter involves blistering followed by desquamation. Frostbite usually occurs after exposure to extreme cold (below 30°F).

Treatment. Treatment of Raynaud's phenomenon should attack the cause and simultaneously support the patient with reassurance and preventative advice. Nicotine is a definite activator and smoking must be eliminated. In inclement weather, warm clothing and gloves must be worn. Holding cold or icy objects must be avoided.

Biofeedback has been effective in many patients. Medical therapy merits evaluation. Tolazoline (Priscoline) gives only temporary relief. Beta blockers have advocates. In severe cases sympathectomies are considered.

In frostbite, the part must be thawed immediately by immersion in a water bath of 104° to 109°F. When a water bath is unavailable, the hands can be placed under the clothing into the opposing axilla. The frostbitten hand must never be rubbed vigorously, nor be covered with snow or ice, as is often recommended.

Second degree frostbite with the formation of blisters, which are considered to be caused by the formation of ice crystals, must not be thawed in the field where they occurred, since reformation is possible. General body temperature must be raised, but artificial vasodilators such as ingested alcohol are ineffectual.

Occlusive Vascular Disease

Vascular impairment may decrease the distal extremity arterial circulation with dire results. These impairments can be a result of rheumatic disease, post-traumatic arteriovenous abnormalities, thrombi, or arteriosclerotic sequelae. Upon detection, arteriography or angiography are indicated, as is surgical intervention.

Compression syndromes have been discussed in Chapter 2.[73]

Volkmann's Ischemic Contracture

This contracture results from vascular occlusion at the level of the elbow or forearm and may be the result of an improper cast, a fracture, hematomas from a penetrating wound, prolonged abnormal pressure from an inappropriate position, or prolonged application of a tourniquet.

Due to its anatomical structure, the flexor compartment of the forearm cannot expand when there is an increase in internal pressure. All the fascial sheaths are tightly attached to bone and allow no expansion.

Onset of a compression compartment syndrome is catastrophic, with sudden, local, painful swelling and tenderness of the forearm and discoloration of the distal hand and fingers. Pulsations of the distal arteries are absent. Movement of the wrist and fingers is passively and actively diminished.

Persistence of this pressure leads to necrosis of the flexors of the wrist and fingers. The extensors are usually spared. The median and ulnar nerves are usually involved, whereas the radial nerve is spared.

The deformities that result from the ischemic necrosis of the compartment muscles are those of unopposed extension from flexor atrophy and contracture. Besides atrophy of the forearm, a typical median-ulnar nerve hand results.

Treatment is preventative. The causative agent must be identified and removed. When circulation is compromised, release of the pressure must be initiated immediately. Splitting of the fascia along the entire length of the involved muscle(s) must be undertaken. The compartment must remain open until circulation is considered to be resumed and then skin grafting can be considered.

Rehabilitation of the hand depends upon the extent of the residual deformity and its restoration potential.

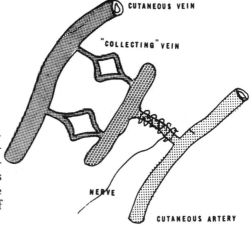

Figure 3–17. Glomus tumor. The tumor is an abnormal connection between a cutaneous artery and vein in which there is swelling and thus irritation of the sensory unmyelinated nerve of the collecting arterioles.

CUTANEOUS VEIN

"COLLECTING" VEIN

NERVE

CUTANEOUS ARTERY

Glomus Tumors

A glomus is a tiny subungual, painful tumor of an arteriovenous anastomosis with an intermediary capillary bed (Fig. 3–17). Its symptoms are pain, tenderness, and sensitivity to external temperature changes—to cold more than heat. The pain is described as sharp and lancing.

The glomus becomes visible or palpable only after a long time, so symptoms may be present long before the diagnosis becomes evident. The tumor begins as a blue spot in the subungual region.

Treatment consists of complete surgical removal, meaning that the entire nail may need to be excised, with the glomus removed down to the bleeding bone.

REFERENCES

1. Pecina MM, Krmpotic-Nemanic J, Markiewitz AD: Tunnel Syndromes. CRC Press, Boca Raton, Fla, 1991.
2. Bonica JJ: The Management of Pain. Lea & Febiger, Philadelphia, 1953.
3. Mitchell SW, Morehouse GR, Keen WW: Gunshot Wounds and Other Injuries of Nerves. JB Lippincott, Philadelphia, 1864.
4. Mitchell SW: Injuries of Nerves and Their Consequences. Smith Elder, London, 1872.
5. Letievant E: Traite de sections nerveuse. JB Bailliere et fils, Paris, France, 1873.
6. Leriche R: De la causalgie envisagee comme une nevrite du sympathique et son traitment par la denudation et l'escision des plexus nerveux periarteriees. Presse Med 24:178–180, 1916.
7. Walker AE, Nulsen F: Electrical stimulation of the upper thoracic portion of the sympathetic chain in man. Arch Neurol Psychiatr, 59:559–560, 1973.
8. Bonica JJ: Causalgic and other reflex sympathetic dystrophies. In Bonica JJ, Liebeskind JC, Albe-Fessard D (eds): Advances in Pain Research and Therapy, Vol 3. Raven Press, New York, 1979, pp 141–166.
9. Merskey H: Development of a universal language of pain syndromes. In Bonica JJ, Lindolom U, Igo A (eds): Advances in Pain Research and Therapy, Vol 5. Raven Press, New York, 1983, pp 37–52.
10. Tahmoush AJ: Causalgia: redefinition as a clinical pain syndrome. Pain 10:187–197, 1981.
11. Hallin RG, Torebjork HE: Observations of hyperalgesia in the causalgia syndrome. Abstract from the Second World Congress on Pain, 1978. In: Rizzi R, Visentin M, Mazzetti G: Reflex Sympathetic Dystrophy: Pain Research and Therapy, Vol 2. Raven Press, New York, 1984.
12. Noordenbos W: Pain. Elsevier/North Holland, Amsterdam, 1959.
13. Devor M: Nerve pathophysiology and mechanisms of pain in causalgia. J Autono Nerv Syst 7:371–384, 1983.
14. Campbell JN, Meyer RA, Raja SN: Is nociceptor activation by alpha-1 adrenoreceptors the culprit in sympathetically maintained pain? APS Journal 1:3–11, 1992.
15. Wall PD, Gutnick M: Ongoing activity in peripheral nerves: the physiology and pharmacology of impulses originating from a neuroma. Exp Neurol 43:580–593, 1974

16. Nathan PW: Involvement of the sympathetic nervous system in pain. In Kosterlitz HW, Terenius LY (eds): Pain and Society. Verlag Chemie, Deerfield Beach, Fla, pp 311–324.

17. Bubusisson D, Fitzgerald M, Wall PD: Ameboid receptive fields of cells in lamina 1, 2 qne 3. Brain Res, 177:376–378, 1979.

18. Cook AJ, Woolf CJ, Wall PD, McMahon SB: Dynamic receptive field plasticity in rat spinal dorsal horn following C-primary afferent input. Nature 325:151–153, 1987.

19. Woolf CJ, Fitzgerald M: The properties of neurones recorded in the superficial dorsal horn in rat spinal cord. J Comp Neurol 221:313–328, 1983.

20. Dubner R: Neuronal plasticity and pain following peripheral tissue inflammation or nerve injury. In Bond MR, Charlton JE, Woolf CJ (eds): Proceedings of the VIth World Congress on Pain. Elsevier, Amsterdam, 1991, pp 263–276.

21. Dubner R, Sharav Y, Gracely RH, Price DD: Ideopathic trigeminal neuralgia: sensory features and pain mechanisms. Pain 31:23–33, 1987.

22. Dubner R, Bennett GJ: Spinal and trigeminal mechanisms of nociception. Ann Rev Neurosci 6:381–418, 1983.

23. Melzack R: Phantom limb pain: implications for treatment of pathological pain. Anesthesiology 35:409–419, 1971.

24. Carron H: Discussion on sympathetic block in pain syndromes. In Rizzi R, Visentin M (eds): Pain Therapy. Elsevier/North Holland, Amsterdam.

25. Roberts WJ: A hypothesis on the physiological basis for causalgia and related pain. Review article. Pain 24:297–311, 1986.

26. Hannington-Kiff JG: Does failed natural opioid modulation in regional sympathetic ganglia cause reflex sympathetic dystrophy: hypothesis. Lancet 338:1125–1127, 1991.

27. Schultzberg M, Hokfelt T, Terenius L, et al: Enkephalin immunoreactive nerve fibers and cell bodies in sympathetic ganglia of the guinea pig and rat. Neuroscience 4:249–270, 1979.

28. Helen P, Panula P, Yang H-YT, Hervonen A, Rappoport SI: Location of substance P, bombesin-gastrin-releasing peptide (Met5) enkephalin and (Met5) enkephalin-Arg4-Phe-like immunoreactivities in adult sympathetic ganglia. Neuroscience 12:907–916, 1984.

29. Thoren P, Floras JS, Hoffman P, Seals DR: Endorphins and exercise: physiological mechanisms and clinical implications. Med Sci Sports Exerc 22:417–428, 1990.

30. Ecker A: Norepinephrine in reflex sympathetic dystrophy: an hypothesis. The Clin J Pain 5:313–315, 1989.

31. VanHoudenhove B: Neuro-algodystrophy: a psychiatrist's view. Clin Rheumatol 5:399–406, 1986.

32. An HS, Hawthorne KB, Jackson WT: Reflex sympathetic dystrophy and cigarette smoking. J Hand Surg 13A:458–460, 1988.

33. Crile GW: The kinetic theory of shock and its prevention through anoci-associated (shockless operation). Lancet 2:7–16, 1913.

34. Hannington-Kiff JG: Analgesia during general anesthesia. Lancet 1:1404–1405, 1988.

35. Ochoa JL: Reflex sympathetic dystrophy: a disease of medical understanding. The Clin J Pain 8:363–366, 1992.

36. Mitchell SW: Injuries of nerves and their consequences. 1872. American Academy of Neurology Reprint Series. Dover, New York, 1965.

37. Livingstone WK: Pain Mechanisms. New York: Macmillan, 1947, pp 209–223.

38. Hannington-Kiff JG: Does failed natural opioid modulation in regional sympathetic ganglia cause reflex sympathetic dystrophy? Lancet 338:1125–1127, 1991.

39. Verdugo R, Ochoa JL: High incidence of placebo responders among chronic neuropathic pain patients. Ann Neurol 30:249, 1991. Abstract.

40. Janig W: Comment on "Reflex sympathetic dystrophy: A disease of medical understanding." The Clin J Pain 8:367–369, 1992.
41. Roberts WJ: Review article: a hypothesis of the physiological basis for causalgia and related pain. Pain 24:300, 1986.
42. Janig W: Experimental approach to reflex sympathetic dystrophy and related syndromes. Pain 46:241–245, 1991.
43. Houdenhove BV, Vasquez G, Onghena P, Stans L, Vandeput C, Vermaut G, Vervaeke G, Igodt P, Vertmmen H: Etiopathogenesis of reflex sympathetic dystrophy: a review and biopsychosocial hypothesis. The Clin J Pain 8:300–306, 1992.
44. Bruehl S, Carlson CR: Predisposing psychological factors in the development of reflex sympathetic dystrophy. A review of the empirical evidence. The Clin J Pain, 8:287–299, 1992.
45. Cailliet R: Reflex sympathetic dystrophy. In Cailliet R: Shoulder Pain, ed 3. FA Davis, Philadelphia 1991, pp 227–252.
46. Kosin F, McCarty DJ, Sims J, Genant H: The reflex sympathetic dystrophy syndrome. Am J Med 60:321–331, 1976.
47. Wang JK, Johnson KA, Ilstrup DM: Sympathetic blocks for reflex sympathetic dystrophy. Pain 23:13–17, 1985.
48. Fields HL: Editorial comment. Pain 49:161–162, 1992.
49. Janig W, Blumberg H, Bas RA, Campbell JA: The reflex sympathetic dystrophy syndrome: consensus statement and general recommendations for diagnosis and clinical research. In Bond MR, Charlton JE, Woolf CJ (eds): Pain research and clinical management: proceedings of the VIth World Congress on Pain, Vol 4. Elsevier, Amsterdam, 372–375, 1991.
50. Janig E: Pathobiology of reflex sympathetic dystrophy: some general considerations. In Stanton-Hicks M, Jang W, Boas RA (eds): Reflex Sympathetic Dystrophy. Kluwer, Boston, 1990, pp 42–54.
51. Evans JA: Reflex sympathetic dystrophy. Surg Gynecol Obstet 82:36–43, 1946.
52. Wall PD, Gutnick M: Ongoing activity in peripheral nerves: the physiology and pharmacology of impulses originating from a neuroma. Exp Neurol 43:580–593, 1974.
53. Tanelian DL, MacIver MB: Analgesic concentrations of lidocaine suppress tonic A-delta and C fiber discharges produced by acute injury. Anaesthesiology 74:934–936, 1991.
54. Rowbotham MC, Reisner-Keller MB, Fields HL: Both intravenous lidocaine and morphine reduce the pain of posttherapeutic neuralgia. Neurology 41:1024–1028, 1991.
55. Price DD, Long S, Huitt C: Sensory testing of pathophysiological mechanisms of pain in patients with reflex sympathetic dystrophy (clinical section). Pain 49:163–173, 1992.
56. Pratt RB, Balter K: Posttraumatic reflex sympathetic dystrophy: mechanisms and medical management. J Occup Rehabil 1:57–70, 1991.
57. Cain HD, Liebgold HB: Compressive centripetal wrapping technic for reduction of edema. Arch Phys Med Rehabil 48:420, 1967.
58. Richlin DM, Carron H, Rowlingson JC, et al: Reflex sympathetic dystrophy: successful treatment by transcutaneous nerve stimulation. J Pediatr 93:84, 1978.
59. Linson MA, Leffert R, Todd DP: The treatment of upper extremity reflex sympathetic dystrophy with prolonged continuous stellate ganglion blockade. J Hand Surg (Am) 8:153–159, 1983.
60. DeTakats G: Sympathetic reflex dystrophy. Med Clin North Am 49:117–129, 1965.
61. Ladd AL, DeHaven KE, Thanik J, Patt RB, Feuerstein M: Reflex sympathetic imbalance: response to epidural blockade. Am J Sports Med 17:660–667, 1989.

62. Dirksen R, Rutgers MJ, Coolen JMW: Cervical epidural steroids in reflex sympathetic dystrophy. Anesthesiology 66:71–73, 1987.
63. Fink BR: History of local anesthesia. In Cousins MJ, Bridenbaugh PO (eds): Neural Blockade. JP Lippincott, Philadelphia, 1980, pp 3–18.
64. Max MB, Culnane M, Scafer SC, et al: Amitriptyline relieves diabetic neuropathy in patients with normal or depressed mood. Neurology 37:589–596, 1987.
65. Talor JC, Brauer S, Espir MLE: Long-term treatment of trigeminal neuralgia with carbamezapine. Postgrad Med J 57:8–16, 1981.
66. Abram SE, Lightfoot RW: Treatment of long-standing causalgia with prazosin. Reg Anaeth 6:79–81, 1981.
67. Simone DA, Ochoa J: Early and late effects of prolonged topical capsaicin on cutaneous sensibility in neurogenic vasodilitation in humans. Pain 47:285–294, 1991.
68. Prough DS, McLeskey CH, Pehling GG, et al: Efficacy of oral nifedipine in the treatment of reflex sympathetic dystrophy. Anaesthesiology 62:796–799, 1985.
69. Cailliet R: Differential diagnosis of neck, arm and hand pain. In Cailliet R: Neck and Arm Pain, ed 3. FA Davis, Philadelphia, 1991, pp 194–220.
70. Buerger L: The Circulatory Disturbances of the Extremities. WB Saunders, Philadelphia, 1924.
71. Miller N: Learning of visceral and glandular responses. Science 163:434–435, 1969.
72. Proctor MR: Biofeedback. In Warfield CA (ed): Manual of Pain Management. JB Lippincott, Philadelphia, 1991.
73. Mabee JR, Bostwick TL: Pathophysiology and mechanisms of compartment syndrome. Orthop Rev 175–181, 1993.

CHAPTER 4

Common Tendinitis Problems of the Hand and Forearm

Trauma to the tendons of the hand is a frequent cause of pain and impairment, yet symptomatic inflammation of the tendons and peritendinous tissues of the body remains poorly understood. The gross and histopathologic changes in these tissues are nonspecific. They include fibrocytic proliferation, thickening, destruction of synovial tissue, and often adhesion to adjacent soft tissues. A diagnosis of tendinitis implies inflammation causing abnormal function of a tendon, with impairment and often pain.

Tendons normally connect muscle to bone for articular function of the extremities, and the muscle tonus generally determines the tension within the tendon fibers. The collagen fibers (Fig. 4–1) that form the tendons have a normal "curled" configuration. The collagen fibril is a crystalline tropocollagen molecule formed by chemically bonded atoms. These fibrils are embedded within a ground substance containing glycosaminoglycans, proteoglycans, and glycoproteins. In a tendon, the collagen fibers lie parallel to each other (Fig. 4–2). In the resting stage of physiologic curl they maintain tone. The tone of the muscle tendon complex mechanism, which determines the tone within the tendon, is determined by the tone of the extrafusal fibers of the muscle (Fig. 4–3).[1] Muscle tone is determined by intrinsic neurologic mechanisms, in which the spindle system feedback operates in conjunction with the Golgi apparatus feedback, within the tendon itself.[1] The spindle system determines the rate of elongation, whereas the Golgi apparatus determines the strength (force) of the contraction. This mechanism has been

160

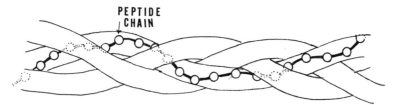

PEPTIDE
CHAIN

Figure 4–1. Tropocollagen trihelix fiber (schematic). This type I collagen molecule is composed of peptide chains composed of two α_1 and one α_2 peptide chains in which every third molecule is a glycine amino acid. The three intertwining peptide chains form a trihelix collagen fiber. (Modified from Alberts B, Bray D, Lewis J, et al: Molecular Biology of the Cell. Garland, New York, 1983, p 694.)

thoroughly discussed in Chapter 2. The force of neuromusculotendinous contractions is measured in newtons.°

The extrafusal muscles contract concentrically and eccentrically causing the tendon fibers to also undergo commensurate tension and elongation. Deceleration of a musculotendinous unit occurs frequently in daily neuromuscular actions, and involves even greater forces than do concentric forces,[2] a fact frequently overlooked in the clinical setting.

The relaxation after a muscular contraction allows the tendon fibrils to recoil. If the contraction is excessive or prolonged, without an interim rest period, the fibrils undergo excessive elongation with some internal structural disruption.

The mechanical behavior of tendons when they are elongated until there is a specific degrees of rupture has been a source of study. Rupture is a break in the peptide chain after a greater than physiologic force of elongation. These forces are plotted in a "stress-strain curve," in which stress is the amount of load per unit cross-sectional area and strain the proportional elongation that results.

Different regions of the tendon that react to elongation forces plotted on the stress-strain curve have been postulated:

The toe region,[3] in which "physiologic" loading occurs for 1 hour.

The linear region, in which the stress increases rapidly and causes prolonged elongation. Microfailure of the tissue results.

°A newton is the force that will give a mass of 1 kilogram an acceleration of 1 meter per second per second. The term "kilopound" is also used.

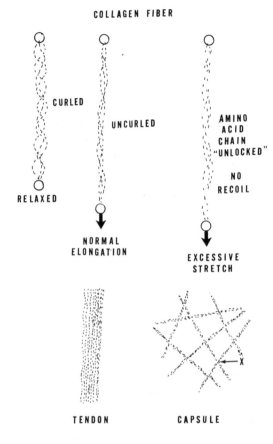

Figure 4-2. Collagen fiber. Each collagen fiber is a tri-helix chain of amino acids bound together chemically (electrically). They uncurl to their physiologic length, then recoil when the elongation force is released. If the collagen fiber is elongated past its physiologic length, the amino acid chains become disrupted, and the fiber no longer returns to its resting length. A tendon consists of parallel bands of collagen fibers. In a capsule, the collagen fibers crisscross and glide over each other at their intersection (X). The capsule depicted here elongates as far as each collagen fiber permits.

The progressive failure region, in which the tendon remains intact to the naked eye but microscopically demonstrates significant failure.

The major failure region, where the tendon still remains "intact" but there are frank ruptures.

The complete rupture region, in which there is gross tendon disruption.[4]

All these "regions" are arbitrary and based on microscopic changes; the value of identifying them lies in their relationship to "recovery." Recovery is the return of the tendon to its original length. The recovery of a tendon after stretch can be beneficially modified by conditioning of the tendon with gentle stretching prior to testing.[3] "Recovery" has unfortunately been used to imply that no permanent damage or permanent elongation remains after stretching; however, microfailure apparently remains.[4,5]

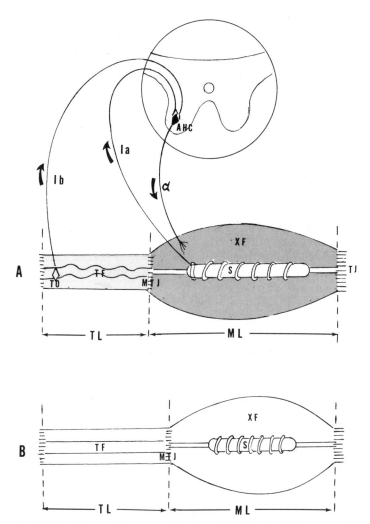

Figure 4–3. Musculo-tendinous mechanism. *(A)* The Spindle system (S) measures the length of the muscle (ML) and the tendon organs (Golgi) (TO) monitor the tension. Stretching of the spindle system activates the Ia fiber whereas stretching the tendon organs activate the IB fibers. These influence the anterior horn cell (AHC), which sends motor fiber activity via the alpha fibers to the extrafusal fibers (XF). With the muscle at resting level (A) the tendon fibers (TF) are slight coiled. When the extrafusal fibers contract *(B)* the muscle shortens (ML), the tendon elongates (TL) to the degree that the tendon fibers can elongate. The tendon fibrills (TF) uncoil. Excessive muscle contraction can tear the muscle-tendon juncture (MJT).

The stress-strain curve depends on many factors besides prestretch conditioning. The rate of stretch has influence on the ultimate recovery.[6] In an ideal spring, elongation is independent of the speed of stretch, with the tension remaining the same over all lengths. Collagen does not perform as an ideal spring. A tendon gradually lengthens from a constant or repeated load. This slow elongation is termed "creep" and is transient if the force is within physiologic limits.

The viscoelastic properties of collagen vary with temperature. A temperature below 37°C can be considered physiologic and there is good recovery from stretch; whereas temperatures between 37° and 40° allow increased creep, and temperatures above 40° contribute to permanent damage by "melting" the bonds between tropocollagen molecules. These factors have clinical significance, since damage and recovery are dependent upon stress and ambient temperature.

There are nontraumatic factors that affect tendons. Immobilization causes significant loss of strength. The dense connective tissue of muscle loses 80 percent of its strength within 4 weeks, that of ligaments loses 50 percent after 8 weeks. In tendons, there is loss in length and flexibility rather than loss of strength.

In their daily function, tendons are subjected to tensile forces, and to compressive and shear stresses.[6] Microfailure occurs if the tendon load is excessive or if the rest between loads is insufficient to allow the tendon fibrils to recover resting length.[7] Repetitive loading stress accelerates the microtrauma, eventually exceeding the reparative capacity of the tendon.[8]

The pathologic changes within the tendon include swelling and thickening of the sheaths; this causes vascular impairment within the mesotendon and failure of the normal diffusion of nutritive elements.[9] (See Fig. 4-4.)

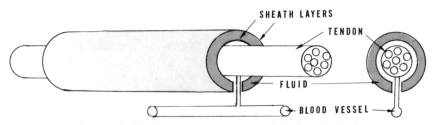

Figure 4-4. Tendon sheaths and blood supply (schematic). Tendons are protected by a sheath that protects them, lubricates and permit nutritional blood supply. The sheath layers are the inner "visceral" and outer "parietal" between which is a thin layer of lubricant resembling synovial fluid. A longitudinal fold permits small blood vessels to enter the sheath.

Tendons glide upon their contiguous tissues. This gliding is facilitated by the thin fibrous and cellular layers of the tendon, known as epitenon, which adhere to the tendon surfaces. The tendons within sheaths contain synovial fluid for lubrication of the tendon inside the sheath, and the sheath has external lubricant at the interface with peritendinous tissues.

The viability and integrity of tendons are affected by systemic factors such as rheumatoid arthritis, hypothyroidism, diabetes mellitus, gout, calcium pyrophosphate deposits, collagen vascular disease, and infections.[10]

Occupational stress factors are frequently the cause of tendinitis. These are termed cumulative trauma disorders (CTS), and result from repetitive tasks requiring forceful motions, unusual postures, exposure to temperature extremes, and exposure to vibration.[11] These factors were recognized as early as 1717.[12]

Diagnostic examination reveals swelling, tenderness, warmth, crepitus, snapping, and occasionally numbness. Direct identification of the involved tendon is necessary, and placing that specific tendon under stress (resisted movement) or passive elongation reveals the precise tendon affected.

Every tendon in the hand is a potential site of tendonitis. Most sites can be isolated by evaluating the specific functional impairment of that precise tendon.

TENDON RUPTURE

A tendon may be ruptured from an acute stretch injury when the fibrils are elongated beyond their physiologic recoil. The tendon is normally strongest at its musculotendinous link, where it seldom tears. Tearing does occur at its insertion site, with or without avulsion of the bone or periosteum. A tendon involved in systemic disease or a tendon that has sustained numerous microtraumata will more frequently tear from a relatively low stress.

Precise anatomical sites of hand-finger tendon injuries will be discussed.

Extensor Tendons

Injury to extensor tendons of the fingers and thumb is common, as they are superficially prominent and have little overlying skin and subcutaneous tissue as protection. They are also subject to direct injury when the hand and fingers are in the extended position. A thorough knowledge of functional anatomy is necessary to accurately diagnose and treat these injuries.

Extensor tendons tend NOT to retract after being severed and thus can be sutured soon after injury. They require 3 to 4 weeks before they regain integrity. Suture material should not be absorbable as integrity, which is usually achieved in 3 weeks, may not be gained by the time of absorption of the suture material.

After approximation and suture during the first 2 to 3 days, there is an outpouring of fibrin, which becomes invaded by fibrobasts within 5 days. These fibrin fibrils fuse into long threads that bridge the gap between the two severed ends. By the third week, edema has usually subsided and excessive vascularity has decreased. The union is, at this time, sufficiently strong to allow some traction upon the tendon.

Tendons contained within a sheath, when severed, show more deterioration and heal more slowly than those not contained within a sheath. The reason is that the swelling of the injured tendon within the sheath obstructs venous and lymphatic return and impairs tendon nutrition and subsequent healing. Adhesions may form about the tendon; these may also impair nutrition and ultimately impair function.

The exact technique of tendon suturing is beyond the scope of this text, but postsuture management needs discussion. Once sutured, the wrist must be immobilized for 3 to 4 weeks with 30° to 40° extension of the fingers. This violates the principal of immobilization in a "position of function," that is, with the wrist slightly extended and the fingers flexed. Fortunately, suturing of extensor tendons usually results in good function in spite of this postoperative immobilization.

The extensor pollicis longus tendon usually retracts a considerable distance and this may present difficulty in locating the proximal end. Search for this portion of the tendon is best achieved through an incision above the wrist, with approximation of the ends by means of a probe.

Due to varying characteristics of extensor tendon anatomy injuries must be so oriented. Zones have been designated (Fig. 4–5).

Flexor Tendons

Suturing a flexor tendon in "no man's land" (Fig. 4–6) has an unfavorable prognosis. The anatomical structure and relationship of the tendons in the area indicate the reason for this poor prognosis. A sutured tendon usually swells, and in this area of the fingers there is no room for expansion of the tendon. Ischemic necrosis can result.

Primary suturing of a flexor tendon within 'no man's land' should be avoided. Primary care should be concerned with the wound, and a tendon transplant should be considered some 4 to 5 weeks later. Pri-

Figure 4-5. Anatomical zones of tendon injuries. Zone I is at the DIP joint level and zone 8 (not shown) is at the distal forearm level. Muscular injuries occur proximal to zone 8 and tendons at zones 7 and 8 are beneath subcutaneous, reticulum and fascial levels. The tendons at zone 6 are very superficial and are relatively round or oval. Lacerations at zone 5 are at the MP joint level. Tendons at this level usually do not retract. Zones 4 and 3 are at the Interphalangeal joint level and rarely include complete lacerations or the dorsal apparatus. Lacerations at zones 2 and 1 are conceptually simple: thin and oriented upon the dorsal aspect of the middle phalanx. The thumb zones (T_I-T_V) are discussed in the text.

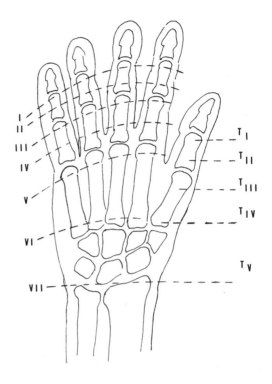

mary suture may be done for tendons severed "distal" to no man's land, that is, profundus tendons. In these severed tendons the distal portion of the profundus tendon can be surgically removed and the proximal end reattached. The resultant shortened tendon does not interfere with the uninjured superficialis function.

Primary suture of severed flexor tendons proximal to no man's land, especially at the wrist level, yields good functional results. Attempting to resuture "individual" tendons, profundus to profundus or superficialis to superficialis, usually results in functional failure. Usually only the profundus tendon is repaired. As this tendon flexes the distal interphalangeal joint, good finger function results.

SPECIFIC TENDINITIS PROBLEMS

Extensor Tendon Tears

Mallet Finger. Tear of the extensor tendon from its attachment on the distal phalanx (Fig. 4-7) usually occurs from an acute flexion injury

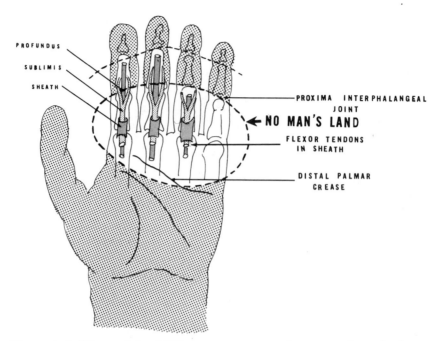

Figure 4–6. "No man's land." This area represents the region where the flexor tendons (profundus and sublimis) are tightly enclosed within a sheath. Primary repair of tendons in this region is *contraindicated*. Suture of the skin should be contemplated. Primary suture between the two interphalangeal joints should be avoided because the tendon inserts in this region.

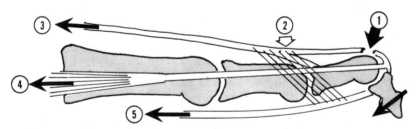

Figure 4–7. Distal phalanx extensor tendon tear (mechanism). The mechanism of the mallet finger is described. The arrow depicts flexion of the distal phalanx: (1) tear of the extensor tendon upon the distal phalanx; (2) landsmeer ligament that connects the extensor and flexor tendons; (3) extensor tendon pull; (4) lumbrical muscle pull; (5) profundus flexor muscle pull.

to the finger when the extensor tendon is taut. Most cases have the tendon torn from its insertion upon the phalanx, and 25 percent sustain a bone avulsion from the injury.

Conservative treatment consists of immobilization of the distal phalanx in hyperextension (Fig. 4–8) for 5 weeks and usually results in functional recovery. By flexing the middle phalanx and extending the distal phalanx the central extensor slip will pull the extensor mechanism distally and allow the torn tendon to reunite (Fig. 4–9). In this finger position the lateral bands are relaxed. If treatment is begun within 10 days of the injury functional recovery is usually achieved by using a cast (Fig. 4–10) for 5 weeks, followed by splinting the distal phalanx for another 4 weeks. If contracture of the flexors has occurred, passive stretch may be needed as well as gentle active extensor exercises. Surgical intervention is indicated when functional restoration has not been achieved or the resultant function accepted by the patient.

Extensor Tendon Rupture at the Middle Phalanx. Rupture of the insertion of the extensor tendon into the middle phalanx, with or without bony avulsion, may occur from a direct blow or crushing injury. Previous injuries may have permitted attenuation of the tendon that now has ruptured from a lesser force.

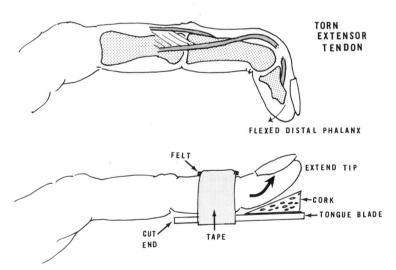

Figure 4–8. Conservative management of the mallet finger. Rupture of the extensor tendon to the distal phalanx results in acute flexion of the finger tip, which cannot be actively extended. Immobilizing the distal phalanx in "hyperextension" for four to five weeks usually allows functional healing. The splint is a tongue blade reaching only to the middle phalangeal joint. The cork is glued to a tongue blade, which extends past the tip of the finger to protect that digit. The felt between the tape protects the dorsum of the finger.

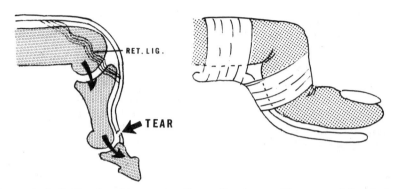

Figure 4–9. Rationale of treatment for mallet finger. Flexing middle phalanx and extending the distal digit permits the extensor tendon to unite. This position pulls the extensor mechanism distally and relaxes the lateral bands.

Rupture of the extensor tendon at that site causes the proximal phalanx to extend and the middle phalanx to flex (Fig. 4–11). This deformity is termed boutonniere deformity and may result from rheumatoid disease and/or trauma. Because of the inadequate extensor slip function, the lateral bands dislocate to the flexor side of the joint fulcrum. This results in a flexion deformity of the proximal interphalangeal joint and hyperextension of the distal joint.

Treatment of this deformity is difficult, as a functional splint (Fig. 4–12) is often ineffective, but a rigid splint may fix the manually corrected deformity (Fig. 4–13).

Extensor Pollicus Longus Rupture. The extensor pollicis longus tendon curves around the dorsal radial tubercle of Lister (Fig. 4–14), passes over the radial wrist extensor, and continues to the thumb. Wear and tear can occur at the point where the tendon angulates. Rupture of this ligament results in the inability to extend the distal joint of the thumb and in weakness in extending the proximal joint. Normally the tendon can be palpated when the wrist is actively extended and the thumb abducted.

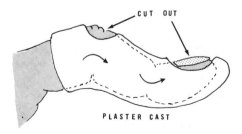

Figure 4–10. Plaster cast treatment for mallet finger. The cast holds the distal joint hyperextended and the middle joint flexed. The dorsum of the middle joint and the nail are exposed.

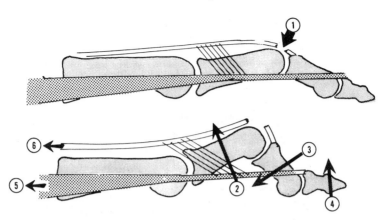

Figure 4–11. Boutonniere deformity: tear of extensor tendon slip (mechanism). When there occurs a tear (1) of the central slip of the extensor tendon the lateral bands (2) migrate volarly from contraction of the extensor tendon (6), the intrinsics (5) contract and flex the proximal interphalangeal joint (3). The distal phalanx extends (4).

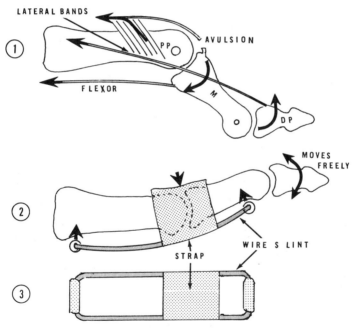

Figure 4–12. Buttonhole rupture, extensor tendon at middle joint, split treatment. (1) Avulsion of the extensor tendon permits the lateral bands to move in a palmar direction, pulling in a proximal direction. The flexor tendons now flex the middle phalanx (MP) and the lateral bands extend the distal phalanx (DP). (2) The splint is made of firm wire bent to extend the middle joint. The strap is inelastic. The distal phalanx is left free and motion is encouraged. (3) Dorsal view of the splint.

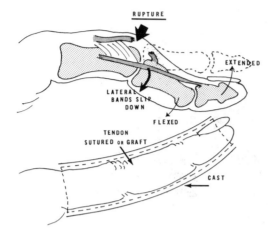

Figure 4-13. Extensor communis tear, surgical repair followed by plaster splint. The mechanism described in 4-12 is shown. After surgical repair, the finger can be splinted as shown.

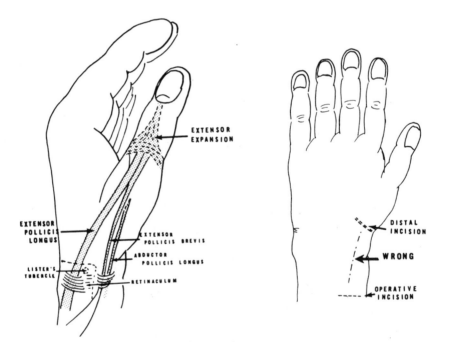

Figure 4-14. Rupture of the extensor pollicis longus. The extensor pollicis longus extends to the distal phalanx along a diagonal course. Its rupture results in loss of extension of the distal digit of the thumb, and some weakness of extension of the proximal joint. The ruptured tendon retracts considerably. End-to-end suture is not feasible, and grafting is required. Rather than extending the laceration, a proximal incision to locate the distal tendon must be made, and the graft is then passed through the canal with a smooth probe.

After rupture, primary suturing of the two fragmented ends of the tendon is not possible, as this repair will neither hold nor function. Repair requires a graft, extending from a site proximal to the dorsal retinaculum to the end located at the metacarpal. Repair may necessitate the transfer of the tendon of the extensor indicis. Once grafted, the thumb needs to be splinted for at least 1 month before use.

Tendinitis of the Extensor Compartments

De Quervain's Disease. Tenosynovitis of the thumb abductors at their radiostyloid process caused by stenosis is very common. The condition was named after the Swiss surgeon De Quervain.[11] The first dorsal compartment contains the abductor pollicis longus and the extensor pollicis brevis (see Fig. 4–14); it is confined by the radial styloid and covered by a synovially lined ligament 1.5 inches long.[12,13] Numerous structural abnormalities have been described, such as a division into two compartments by a septum (in 21–34% of dissected cases).[14,15]

Symptoms are swelling and pain over the radial styloid, with the pain initiated and aggravated by forcing the wrist into an ulnar deviated position, with the thumb flexed and abducted (Finkelstein's test).[16] Tenderness over the extensor sheath is elicited and often accompanied by swelling and thickness. (Figure 4–15) Occasionally a trigger finger[17] or crepitation[18] may be observed on active extension and passive flexion in the test position. Resistance of thumb abduction may reproduce the symptoms.

De Quervain's disease may be confused with Wartenberg's syndrome, which is a nerve entrapment of the superficial branch of the radial sensory nerve.[19] Wartenberg, in 1932, suggested use of the term "cheirlagia paresthetica"[20] analogy to paresthetica meralgia.[21] This condition usually occurs as a result of trauma, such as surgery for De Quervain's disease, compressive plaster casts, tight wrist cuffs, and so on.

The pathology is increased vascularity of the outer sheath, with edema that thickens the sheath and constricts the enclosed tendon. The synovial fluid tends to increase and thicken, with the formation of fine hairlike fibers that adhere to the adjacent tissues. The tendon and its sheath may increase in thickness to twice the normal size.

The clinical symptoms and signs are subjective paresthesia over the dorsum of the hand, with objective hypesthesia to sensory testing (Fig. 4–16). Pressure or percussion over this branch of the radial nerve at the extensor carpi radialis longus insertion or from "hyper"pronation of the forearm reproduces the patient's symptoms (a positive Tinel sign). There may be a "burning" sensation over the area of hypalgesia, and trophic skin changes when the condition becomes chronic.

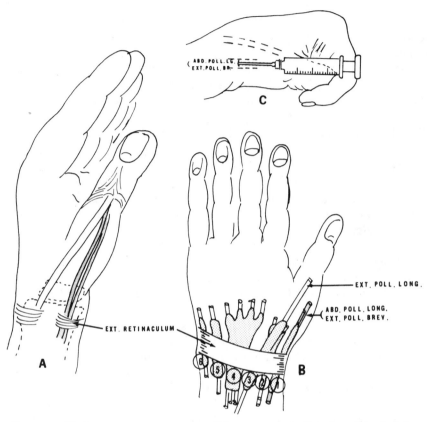

Figure 4–15. Stenosing tenosynovitis of the extensor pollicis brevis and abductor pollicis longus, De Quervain's disease. *(A)* The tendons pass over the prominence of the radial styloid process. The extensor pollicis longus tendon forms the ulnar border of the snuff box. *(B)* The six tendon sheaths pass under the extensor retinaculum. (1) and (3) are labeled, (2) contains the tendon of the extensor carpi radialis, (4) the extensor digitorum communis, (5) the extensor digit minimi, and (6) the extensor carpi ulnaris. Tenosynovitis occurs commonly only at (1). *(C)* Method and site of injection of steroids in this condition.

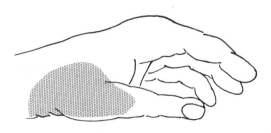

Figure 4–16. Dermatome area of the superficial branch of the radial nerve.

Damage to this branch of the radial nerve can cause functional impairment if it occurs in the dominant hand.

Treatment. For De Quervain's disease, splinting of the thumb and oral anti-inflammatory medication can be tried, but local injection of steroids is preferable, as one injection often suffices.[14] Accurate technique is critical. The needle is inserted into the distal end of the compartment and the gradual swelling from the anesthetic agent confirms its entry into the compartment.[15]

In resistant cases, surgical release may be required, although results have been disappointing.[22] The surgical techniques are beyond the scope of this text, but it may be stated that incisions must not be longitudinal along the tendon sheath, as this type of incision tends to scar or even form keloid. A transverse incision undermining the skin, followed by longitudinal incision of the overlying fascia and sheath will decompress the tendon.

Wartenberg's syndrome is best treated with local application of corticosteroid ointments or histamine by iontophoresis. If conservative treatment fails, surgical exploration may be necessary.

Extensor Pollicis Longus Tendinitis

Stenosing tenosynovitis of the extensor pollicis longus tendon (EPL) may occur when the EPL muscle extends into a tight third compartment. This condition constricts normal thumb flexion and causes pain, tenderness, swelling, and crepitation at Lister's tubercle.

Attrition and even rupture of the EPL tendon may occur when splints and noninflammatory medications fail and are more probable after frequent steroid injections.[23,24] They may be obviated by rerouting the tendon.

Extensor Indicis Proprius Syndrome

The extensor indicis proprius (EIP) muscle belly often lies within the fourth dorsal compartment.[25] Swelling and/or hypertrophy from repetitive exercises may cause (Fig. 4–17) synovitis with resultant stenosis. Clinically there is localized pain, from resistance to index finger extension while holding the wrist in a flexed position.

Treatment consists of splinting the wrist in a neutral position with the metacarpophalangeal joints in slight extension. Oral anti-inflammatory medication is usually effective, as are local injections of anesthetic agents and steroids. In persistent cases, surgical release of the compartment affords relief.

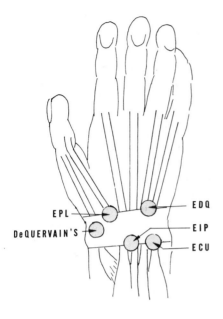

Figure 4–17. Tendinitis sites on dorsum of the wrist extensor tendons. EPI = extensor pollicis longus tendon; EIP = extensor indicis proprius tendon; EDQ = extensor digiti quinti tendon; ECU = extensor carpi ulnaris tendon.

Extensor Digiti Minimi Tendinitis (EDM)

Swelling and pain on extension of the fifth finger occurs just distal to the ulnar head. Stenosis occurs rarely.

Local splinting and injections under the slip are usually effective.

Extensor Carpi Ulnaris Tendinitis

Tendinitis of the extensor carpi ulnaris (ECU) is a tenosynovitis of the sixth dorsal compartment.[26] Subluxation of the tendon may result from a tear in the retinacular ulnar compartment.[27] The subluxation is caused by the patient's actively supinating the hand with the wrist in ulnar deviation. It is reduced by pronating the hand in a radial direction.

Initial treatment is to splint the wrist in extension pronation and radial deviated position plus anti-inflammatory medication. If the subluxation persists, surgical intervention is indicated.[28]

Tendinitis in the Flexor Compartments

Trigger Fingers. Snapping of the flexor tendons during active finger flexion is termed "trigger fingers" and may be felt and be audible

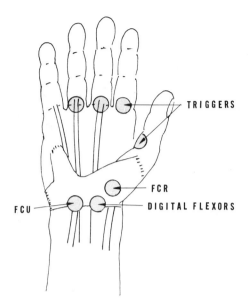

Figure 4–18. Flexor sites of tendinitis (palmar view). Depicts the common location of flexor tendinitis in the palmar aspect of the wrist and fingers.

in the act of flexing and/or re-extension. Flexion is restricted; then, as flexion is further attempted, there is sudden flexion. Once flexed the finger remains locked in the flexed position and cannot be re-extended.

The trigger action occurs most frequently in the middle or ring finger, and is related to direct, repetitive trauma to the flexor tendons of the fingers (Fig. 4–18). As a result of trauma the ligamentous sheath thickens (Fig. 4–19). The enclosed tendon enlarges into a fusiform swelling and forms a nodule within the thickened synovium-lined sheath. When the nodule has passed the annular ligament, the finger has "snapped" and remains flexed. The opposite occurs during active or passive extension. The nodule moves within the ligamentous sheath until the nodule becomes so thick or the sheath so constricted that obstruction occurs. At this point "snapping" ceases and the tendon becomes blocked being able neither to flex nor to extend.

Treatment consists of injecting a steroid within the sheath to expand the constricted sheath. The nodule remains but may now be able to pass the previous obstruction. Failure of this procedure prompts surgical intervention, in which a transverse incision of the sheath proximal to the nodule exposes the annular band, which is slit. Excision of the nodule invariably causes formation of a new and often bigger nodule.

Flexor Carpi Ulnaris Tendinitis

Tendinitis of this tendon (FCU) is common and results from repetitive trauma. It is especially common in tennis players or carpenters.

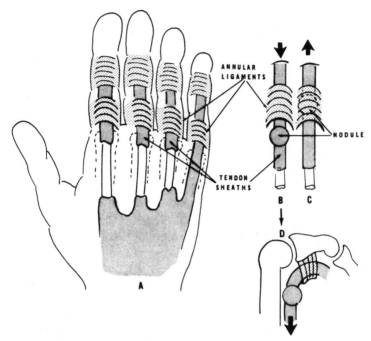

Figure 4–19. Trigger fingers (flexor tendinitis). Depicts the anatomy of the flexor tendons. *(A)* The flexor tendons within their synovial sheaths as they pass under the annular ligament at the metacarpal heads. *(B)* The fusiform swelling of the tendon plus thickening of the sheath proximal to the ligament. *(C)* The nodule permits extension of the finger by passing under the ligament. In *(D)* extension is prevented as the nodule is too large to pass under the ligament.

Clinically there is pain and swelling proximal to the pisiform bone. The symptoms are exacerbated by wrist flexion in an ulnar direction. Due to its proximity there may be concurrent compression of the ulnar nerve within Guyon's canal (see Fig. 2–59). Differentiation of tendinitis located in this region from a pisiform fracture or arthritis of that bone can be achieved by reproducing the pain with side-to-side motion of the bone.

Treatment consists of splinting in a mild wrist flexion, oral steroid or nonsteroidal medication, or by direct injection of steroid into the area. In resistant cases, the ligament can be lengthened[29] or the pisiform bone excised.[30]

Flexor Carpi Radialis Tendinitis

When there is synovitis and stenosis of the carpi radialis tendon (FCR) within the transverse metacarpal ligament, there occurs local tenderness, swelling, and pain upon active/resisted wrist flexion in the radial direction. A trigger nodule may occur in this tendon and cause limited wrist radial flexion with snapping.

Conservative treatment is usually ineffectual, and when the condition is disabling surgery is indicated.[31]

Digital Flexor Tendinitis (With or Without Trigger Nodules)

Finger flexor tendinitis may be painful on active finger flexion activities and is often associated with carpal tunnel syndrome (see Fig. 2–54). There may be swelling and palpable crepitus proximal to the wrist flexor crease, with "triggering" at the level of the transverse carpal ligament.[32]

Painful snapping of these tendons is due to a disproportion between the flexor tendon and its sheath,[33,34] with the constriction occurring at the metacarpal head level at the "pulley" (see Fig. 1–62).

Treatment by a single steroid injection is effective in 77 percent of cases, while 28 percent require a second injection.[34] Concurrent splinting for 4 to 6 weeks has its exponents. Spontaneous resolution has been reported.[35] Resistant and disabling cases may require surgical release,[36] but complications such as painful scarring, nerve injuries, and postoperative bowstringing have to be considered.

Calcific Tendinitis

Some cases of tendinitis proceed to form calcific deposits within the tendon. If there is a concurrent metabolic disease such as hyperparathyroid disease or chronic renal failure, these enhance that possibility. Generally the condition is self-limited, but if this is not the case it may be resolved by appropriate splinting, corticosteroid injections, aspiration, and oral nonsteroidal medications.

Dupuytren's Contracture

Dupuytren's contracture is characterized by fibrous contracture of the palmar fascia with resultant flexion contracture of the fingers at the metacarpophalangeal and proximal interphalangeal joints. This condition was first described by Clive in 1808, but Dupuytren first described an operation for its treatment,[37] and his name was thus associated with the abnormality.

The causative factors remain unknown, but there is a gradual thickening of the palmar fascia. The condition was originally found in Caucasian men in their fifth to seventh decades, but there are numerous cases found in women. There often is no incidence of related vocational traumata yet repeated trauma has been implicated.[38] The original association with epilepsy, chronic alcoholism, and pulmonary tuberculosis[37] is no longer considered pertinent.

The palmar fascia (Figs. 1–62 and 1–63) has been described. It covers the palm of the hand; extending proximally as a continuation of the palmaris longus tendon, it proceeds distally into the fingers and ultimately attaches to the sides of the proximal and middle phalanges. The overlying skin is firmly attached to the fascia by numerous fasciculi and there is scant subcutaneous fat (Fig. 4–20). The undersurface tissue

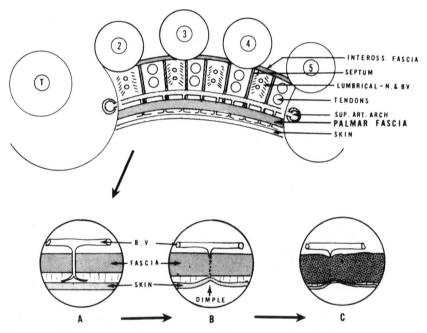

Figure 4–20. Dupuytren's contracture. The upper picture shows the normal anatomy of the palmar fascia. The palmar skin is firmly attached with little subcutaneous fat. Fibrous septa penetrate to the deep interosseous fascia and form spaces. These eight compartments contain the flexor tendons with the alternate compartments containing the lumbrical muscles and neurovascular elements. The skin receives its blood supply by vessels from the superficial arch which penetrates through the fascia. (A) An enlargement of the normal palm (B) Thickening of the fascia constricting the penetrating nutrient artery. The skin puckers to form the characteristic dimple. (C) The fascia ultimately becomes markedly thickened and contracted and the overlying skin atrophic.

of the fascia proceeds into the deeper aspect of the palm along perpendicular fibrous septa. These septa form eight longitudinal compartments, which contain the flexor tendons, their neurovascular bundles, and the lumbrical muscles.

The palmar skin receives its circulation from tiny branches of the superficial volar arch of the radial and ulnar arteries, which penetrate the palmar fascia.

As the fascia undergoes fibrosis, it thickens and contracts, pulls upon the tiny fasciculi connected to the skin, and causes a "dimple" to occur. As the fascia further thickens, it occludes the circulation and causes atrophy of the skin. This progressive ischemia portends poor healing when surgical intervention is contemplated.

The palmar fascial thickening also involves the perpendicular septa and, more distally, the longitudinal bands that pass over the metacarpal heads and attach to the bases of the phalanges. Nodules form in the fascia and the finger flexors develop contractures (Fig. 4–21). These

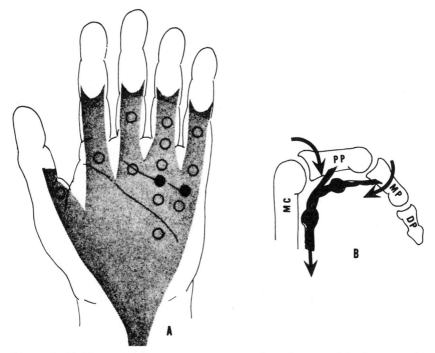

Figure 4–21. Dupuytren's contracture, site and mechanism. (A) These are the principal sites where nodules form in the palmar fascia. The fourth and fifth fingers are most frequently involved. (B) The fascial slips extend to the second phalanx (MP). When they shorten because of contracture, they cause flexion deformity of the metacarpophalangeal or proximal interphalangeal joints, or both.

finger contractures constitute the impairment of Dupuytren's disease. As the fingers attempt to extend in daily activities or from stretching treatment the fascia undergoes further stretching and further hypertrophy.

Symptoms of Dupuytren's contracture are usually a painless thickening of the palmar skin and underlying fascia with some dimpling and palpable nodules. The initial site is usually near the distal palmar crease, with the ring and little finger the most common site. This condition is often unilateral but 40 percent of cases are bilateral.[39] Flexion contractures occur at the metacarpophalangeal joints and cause an inability to fully extend the digits. Pain is rarely, if ever, noted.

A classification of the disease has been offered.[40]

Stage 1: A nodule of the palmar fascia that does not yet include the skin, with no change in the fascia.

Stage 2: A nodule in the fascia with involvement of the skin.

Stage 3. Same as stage 2, but with a flexion contracture of one or more fingers.

Stage 4. Same as stage 3, plus tendon and joint contractures.

Since continued extensor stress upon the hypertrophying fascia causes progression of the syndrome,[41] release of the mechanical stress is the objective of therapy. Release may be simply accomplished by merely excising the fascial and skin bands with a graft insertion.[42] The fascia incised is limited to the palmar fascia and the involved digit.

Preservation of blood supply to the skin requires atraumatic dissection; surgery must be performed in a bloodless field, with absolute hemostasis, closure without tension, and early immobilization. Radical excisions are effective, with a low rate of recurrence; however, the hand may lose as much as 25 percent of its grip power.[43]

Nonsurgical intervention consists of injection of trypsin, chymotrypsin A, hyaluronidase, and lidocaine, followed by gentle yet forceful extension of the fingers.[44] Vitamin E (tocopherol 200 mg daily) has its advocates.[45] These procedures may ultimately insure adequate finger range of motion and are indicated in elderly patients who are either insufficiently impaired to mandate surgical intervention or insufficiently fit to benefit from it. The clinical picture develops at varying speeds, with some cases not progressing over 20 to 30 years. In many cases, this justifies continued observation with no or minimal treatment.

Elbow Pain

Tendinitis. Tendinitis of the wrist and hand has already been discussed, but tendinitis of the elbow is also common and often impairs the patient's ability to work and enjoy athletic activities. The diagnosis of "tendinitis" is often difficult, as findings are subtle.[46] As has been stated, the cause of symptomatic inflammation of tendons and peritendinous tissues of the upper extremity is poorly understood. Often the pathomechanics leading to the inflammation are unclear.[47,48]

Lateral Epicondylitis. Lateral epicondylitis, commonly called "tennis elbow," is a prevalent disorder. Discussion of this condition as a related hand problem is indicated, since the hand muscles (the extensor indicis, extensor carpi ulnaris, extensor digiti minimi, and extensor digitorum communis [Fig. 4–22]) all originate at the elbow (Fig. 4–23). Hand, wrist, and finger extension function initiate, aggravate, and foment this pathologic elbow state.

The condition was originally described, in 1873,[49] as "writer's cramp," and opinions on its etiology and management have varied since. Its incidence in the population varies from 1 to 3 percent. Surprisingly, it is not prominent among manual workers, but is very prominent among recreational tennis players.[50] A similar syndrome on the medial side of the elbow termed "golfer's elbow" is neither as prevalent nor as disabling.[51]

There are three main theories of etiology:

1. Tendinitis of the insertion (origin) at the lateral epicondyle.
2. Entrapment of the radial nerve (Fig. 4–24).
3. Intra-articular or osseous disorders.[52]

Of the tendons involved, the extensor carpi radialis brevis, which inserts (originates) from the lateral epicondyle and the orbicular ligament, has been considered most important.[53] Compression of the radial and posterior osseous nerves (Fig. 4–25) in the radial canal by the fibrous arch of the supinator muscle has been considered a major cause.[54] The extensor carpi radialis brevis and the superficial aspect of the supinator merge at their origin at the lateral epicondyle (Fig. 4–26).

Electromyographic studies to confirm nerve compression have been inconclusive,[55,56] but as several nerves to the elbow were later described (nervus cutaneous antebrachii dorsalis, nervus ramus muscularis anconei, and the periosteal branch),[56] it was recommended that infiltration of these nerves with an anesthetic agent precede any surgical nerve intervention.[57]

Degeneration of the orbicular ligament from overuse can cause chronic impingement of the nerves. In older patients there appear numerous degenerative changes of connective tissue and tendons,[58] and this pattern supports the insertion tendonitis concept of lateral epicondylitis. Surgery to relieve intractable epicondylitis has not proved com-

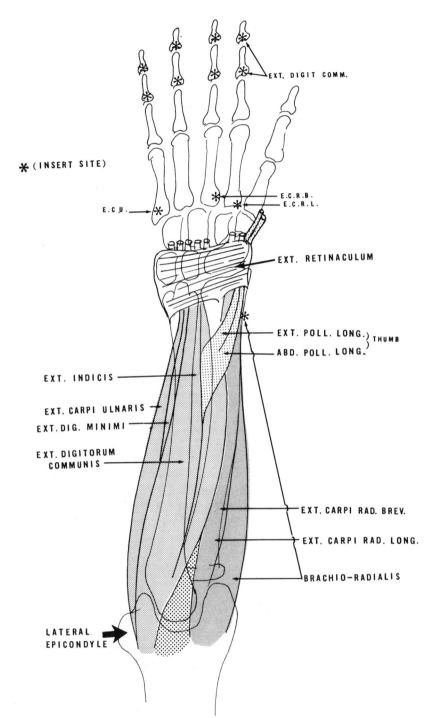

(INSERT SITE) *

EXT. DIGIT COMM.

E.C.R.B.
E.C.R.L.

E.C.U.

EXT. RETINACULUM

EXT. POLL. LONG.) THUMB
ABD. POLL. LONG.

EXT. INDICIS

EXT. CARPI ULNARIS
EXT. DIG. MINIMI

EXT. DIGITORUM
COMMUNIS

EXT. CARPI RAD. BREV.

EXT. CARPI RAD. LONG.

BRACHIO-RADIALIS

LATERAL
EPICONDYLE

Figure 4–22. Extensor muscles of the forearm. The origin and insertion of the extensor muscles are shown as viewed in the left arm and hand. The extensor groups comprise superficial and deep layers which are divided by the extrinsic thumb muscles.

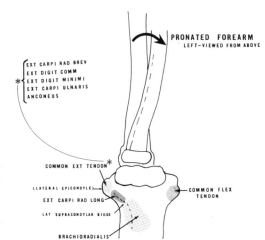

Figure 4–23. Origin of muscles about the elbow. The common extensor tendon originates from the lateral humeral epicondyle. The view presented is the pronated left elbow seen from above.

pletely successful and should thus be considered only after test injections with anesthetic agents.

Clinical Evaluation. The symptoms, an ache and deep tenderness on the extensor aspect of the forearm, locate for the examiner the site of pathology. The origin of the extensor musculature of the hand and fingers at the lateral epicondyle is painful on palpation.

- Resisted wrist extension and radial deviation intensify the pain.
- Resisting supination with the wrist in extension causes tenderness in the area of the posterior interosseus nerve. (See Fig. 4–25).

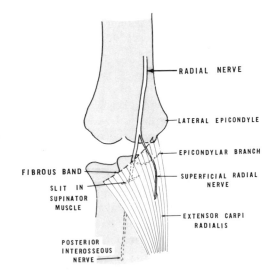

Figure 4–24. Site of muscular attachment at the lateral epicondyle. The muscles that attach from the lateral epicondyle include: (1) extensor indicis; (2) extensor carpi ulnaris; (3) extensor digiti minimi; (4) extensor digitorum communis. Resisting any or all of these muscles can elicit tendinitis at the lateral epicondyle ("tennis elbow").

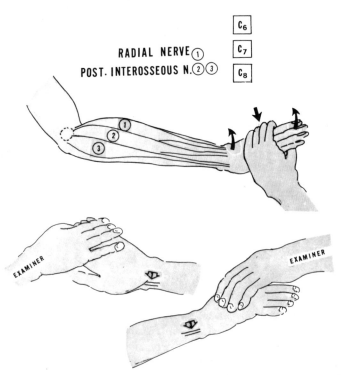

Figure 4-25. Extensor carpi radialis, extensor digitorum communis, and extensor carpi ulnaris. All these muscles originate from the epicondylar area of the humerus. (1) The extensor carpi radialis attaches with the brevis to the bases of the second and third metacarpals (see Fig. 4-22). They are pure wrist muscles and dorsiflex the wrist in a radial direction. (2) The extensor digitorum communis is depicted in 4-22. (3) The extensor carpi ulnaris originates from the lateral epicondyle of the humerus and inserts upon the dorsal surface of the fifth metacarpal. It dorsiflexes the wrist in an ulnar direction.

- Supination places traction upon the annular ligament, and placing resistance upon the extensor carpi radialis brevis (ECRB) implicates its origin as being at the epicondyle.

Treatment

Acute. At its onset, treatment should consist of avoiding those activities of the wrist and hand that cause the pain. Rest of the part implies avoiding wrist and finger extension, and forearm pronation. Local application of ice packs for periods of 20 to 30 minutes several times daily are advisable. Systemic NSAID medication, if tolerated, enjoys support.

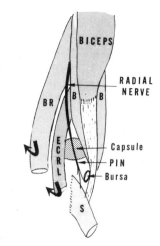

Figure 4-26. Radial nerve at the elbow. The course of the radial nerve at the elbow joint is depicted. B = brachialis muscle; BR = brachioradialis muscle; ECRL = extensor carpi radialis longus; S = supinator muscle; PIN = posterior interosseous nerve. The capsule is that of the elbow joint.

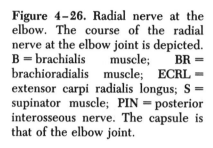

Local rest of the elbow may require splinting of the wrist to prevent or minimize extension. The splint should be worn at night, as well as during the day, for a period of several weeks before it can be considered ineffective. The protective splint should maintain the wrist in 20° of extension, which relieves tension upon the extensor musculature and tendons. Total immobilization of all motions of the elbow must be avoided as this may lead to contracture and so to impairment of all elbow motions.

Modifying activities of daily living should be addressed by teaching the patient to lift objects with the forearm supinated rather than pronated. In athletic activities, changing the style of playing and the equipment may be valid, for example, using a different tennis racquet, two-handed backhand swing, and so on.

Usually the acute symptoms subside within 3 days and local heat can then be used to accelerate healing. A forearm compressive band affords relief while healing occurs. Local injection of steroids is indicated both for differential diagnosis as to the precise pathologic cause, and for treatment. Local anesthetic injection has been considered less effective than steroid injection.[59] Hydrocortisone (25 mg) or triamcinolone (10 mg) is advocated. The patient receiving the injection unfortunately experiences an aggravation of the pain immediately after the injection. This can be minimized if local ice application follows the injection. Conservative management must accompany the injections, and it is possible that this management is more effective than the injections themselves.[60] Acupuncture has actually been claimed to be more effective than injected steroids.[61]

Healing can be considered to have occurred after 6 weeks, and postacute management now must be addressed.

Postacute Management. While the arm is splinted, the patient should not feel pain. Pain at the end range of motion of the wrist and elbow may still persist, but gentle range of motion active and passive exercises should be initiated.

Gentle wrist extensor exercises can be started, with the forearm on a table and the hand extended over the edge (Fig. 4–27). Extensor exercises should include radial and ulnar deviation, both in pronation and supination. Wrist flexion and circumduction should be included. *A period of relaxation MUST follow every period of active exercise.*

When these range of motion exercises can be done without pain, gentle progressive resistance should be initiated, beginning with 1-pound weights and increasing gradually. The weight and repetitions should be gradually increased to the tolerance of the patient.

Activities of daily living, including vocational and sports activities, should be evaluated and modified as indicated.

Surgical Intervention. As a final resort, when symptoms persist, surgical intervention may need to be considered. These procedures vary, and include detachment of the extensor muscle group at the lateral humeral epicondyle, Z lengthening of the extensor carpi radialis

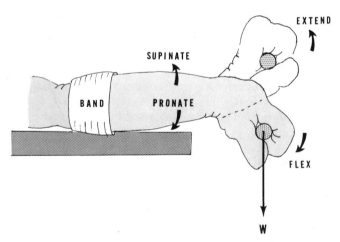

Figure 4–27. Exercises for tennis elbow rehabilitation. With the wrist extended over the edge of a table the flexed hand extends and flexes in degrees of supination and pronation. Done in series with periods of rest the exercise is performed at first without any weight (W) then gradually the weight is increased from one pound to whatever is tolerated. The forearm band is optional but is usually beneficial.

brevis tendon, excision of the annular ligament, excision of the bursa if found enlarged and thickened, and excision of synovial fringes. Techniques and indications are in the realm of the surgeon's experience and are beyond the scope of this text.

Surgical failures include resection of too much annular ligament, which causes instability, inadequate identification and thus inadequate resection of pathologic tissue, and failure to release entrapped nerves.[62]

GENERAL CONCLUSIONS REGARDING TENDON HEALING

In reviewing the recovery of tendinous tissues (generally considered "dense connective tissue") there are several general principles that need to be considered in prescribing treatment and management.

The building block of the tendon is the tropocollagen molecule, which has been described. This ground substance contributes to the tendon's stability and strength. Physical stress influences its organization and reorganization. Creep and recovery depend upon external forces and temperature variations.

The body's repair of tendon damage depends on the vascular status and force of applications. Immobilization causes significant loss of dense connective tissue strength; thus avoidance of excessive immobilization must be observed in all tendon injuries. Immobilization also causes loss of length and flexibility, albeit more slowly than it causes loss of strength.

Treatment of tendon injuries must involve the length of the tendon maintained and the external forces imposed during healing, and the time of immobilization should be carefully considered. The intensities of heat and cold application must be carefully controlled. Early strengthening exercises must be emphasized, and functional restoration must be a foremost consideration in treatment protocols.

Tendon injuries heal in well-established stages. The initial healing stage is that of inflammation, in which vascular cells migrate into the damaged area and bring in fibroblasts, which are the forerunners of ultimate collagen formation. A "neoangiogensis" occurs, in which new blood vessels precede the entry of fibroblasts (fibroplasia). Formation of the fibroblasts is called "fibrillogenesis." This process insures that the ultimate fibers are properly aligned as well as being formed. These healing forces are vascular and stress-related and can be modified by the treatment implied.

These stages are well documented in the literature.[7,63,64]

REFERENCES

1. Dudel J: Muscle. In Schmidt RF (ed): Fundamentals of Neurophysiology, ed 3. Springer-Verlag, New York, 1985, pp 136.
2. Seliger V, Dolejs L, Karas V: A dynamic comparison of maximum eccentric, concentric and isometric contractions using EMG and energy expenditure measurements. Eur J Appl Physiol 45:235–244, 1980.
3. Rigby BJ, Horai N, Spikes JD: The mechanical behavior of rat tail tendon. J Gen Physiol 43:265–283, 1959.
4. Lehman JF, Masock AJ, Warren CG, et al.: Effect of therapeutic temperatures on tendon extensibility. Arch Phys Med Rehabil 50:481–487, 1970.
5. Warren CG, Lehman JF, Koblanski JN: Elongation of rat tail tendon: effect of load and temperature. Arch Phys Med Rehabil 52:465–484, 1971.
6. Van Brocklin JD, Ellis DG: A study of the mechanical behavior of toe extensor tendons under applied stress. Arch Phys Med Rehabil 46:369–370, 1965.
7. Tillman LJ, Cummings GS: Biologic mechanisms of connective tissue mutability. In Currier DP, Nelson RM (eds): Dynamics of Human Biologic Tissues. FA Davis, Philadelphia, 1992, pp 1–44.
8. Armstrong TJ: Ergonomics and cumulative trauma disorders. Hand Clin 2:553, 1986.
9. Goldstein SA, Armstrong TJ, Chaffin DB: Analysis of cumulative strain in tendons and tendonsheaths. J Biomech 20:1, 1987.
10. Manske PR, Ogata K, Lesker PA: Nutrient pathways to extensor tendons of primates. J Hand Surg 10B:8, 1985.
11. deQuervain F: Korresp Bl. Schweiz Arz 25:389, 1895.
12. Lipscomb PR: Tenosynovitis of the hand and wrist: carpal tunnel syndrome, deQuervain's disease, trigger digit. Clin Orthop 13:164, 1959.
13. Lipscomb PR: Stenosing tenosynovitis at the radial styloid process. Ann Surg 134:110, 1951.
14. Harvey FJ, Harvey PM, Horsley MW: DeQuervain's disease: surgical or nonsurgical treatment. J Hand Surg (Am) 15A:83, 1990.
15. Leslie BM, Ericson WB, Morhead JR: Incidence of a septum within the first dorsal compartment of the wrist. J Hand Surg (Am) 15A:88, 1990.
16. Finkelstein H: Stenosing tenosynovaginitis at the radial styloid process. J Bone Joint Surg (Am) 12A:509, 1930.
17. Viegas SF: Trigger thumb of deQuervain's disease. J Hand Surg (Am) 11A:235, 1986.
18. Grunberg AB, Reagon DS: Pathologic anatomy of the forearm: intersection syndrome. J Hand Surg (Am) 10A:299, 1985.
19. Saplys R, Mackinnon SE, Dellon LA: The relationship between nerve entrapment versus neuroma complications and the misdiagnosis of DeQuervain's disease. Contemp Orthoped 15:51, 1987.
20. Wartenberg R: Zach Neurol Psych 141:145, 1932.
21. Pecina MM, Krmpotic-Nemanic J, Markiewitz AD: Syndrome of the superficial branch of the radial nerve. In: Tunnel Syndromes. CRC Press, Boca Raton, Fla., 1991, pp 79–81.
22. Arons MS: DeQuervain's release in working women: a report of failures, complications and associated diagnoses. J Hand Surg (Am) 12A:540, 1987.
23. Gottlieb NL, Riskin WG: Complications of local corticosteroid injections. JAMA 243:1547, 1980.
24. Fitzgerald RH: Intrasynovial injection of steroids: Uses and abuses. Mayo Clin Proc 51:655–659, 1976.
25. Ritter MA, Inglis AE: The extensor indicis proprius syndrome. J Bone Joint Surg (Am) 51A:1645, 1969.

26. Hajj AA, Wood MB: Stenosing tenosynovitis of the extensor carpi ulnaris. J Hand Surg (Am) 11A:519, 1986.
27. Burkhart SS, Wood MB, Linscheid RL: Posttraumatic recurrent subluxation of the extensor carpi ulnaris tendon. J Hand Surg (Am) 7:1, 1982.
28. Wood MB, Dobyns JH: Sports related extraarticular wrist syndromes. Clin Orthop 202:93, 1986.
29. Phalen GS: The carpal tunnel syndrome. J Bone Joint Surg (Am) 48A:211, 1966.
30. Carroll RE, Coyle MP: Dysfunction of the pisotriquetral joint: treatment by excision of the pisiform. J Hand Surg (Am) 10A:703, 1985.
31. Gabel G, Bishop AT, Wood MB: Surgical anatomy and management of flexor carpi ulnaris tendinitis. American Society for Surgery of the Hand Proceedings, Toronto, 1990.
32. Brown LP, Coulson DB: Triggering at the carpal tunnel with incipient carpal tunnel syndrome. J Bone Joint Surg (Am) 56A:623, 1974.
33. Hueston JT, Wilson WF: The etiology of trigger finger. Hand 4:257, 1972.
34. Kolin-Sorenson V: Treatment of trigger fingers. Acta Orthop Scand 41:428, 1970.
35. Newport ML, Lane LB, Stuchin SA: Treatment of the trigger finger by steroid injection. J Hand Surg (Am) 15A:748, 1990.
36. Lapidus PW: Stenosing tenovaginitis. Surg (Am) Clin North Am 33:1317, 1953.
37. Dupuytren G: Clinical lectures on surgery, delivered at Hotel Dieu in 1832. Translated by A.S. Doane. Collins and Hannay. New York, 1833.
38. Deplas B: Inflammation of palmar aponeurosis in workers mounting and repairing telephone cables. Carch D Mal Profess 7:217–219, 1946.
39. Skoog T: Dupuytren's contracture: with special reference to etiology and improved surgical treatment. Acta Chir Scand (Suppl) 139:1, 1948.
40. Shaw MH. Treatment of Dupuytren's contracture. Br J Plast Surg (Am) 4:218–223, 1951.
41. Rhode CM, Jennings WD: Dupuytren's contracture. Am Surg 33:855, 1967.
42. Bassot J: Traitment de las maladie de Dupuytren par exercise pharmaco-dynamic base physiologique technique. Gaz Hop 16:557, 1969.
43. Gordon S: Dupuytren's contracture. Can Med Assoc J 58:543–547, 1948.
44. Byrne JJ: Fibrous hyperplasia. In: The Hand: Its Anatomy and Diseases. Charles C Thomas, Springfield, Ill., 1959, pp 218–236.
45. Steinberg CL: Tocopherols in treatment of primary fibrosis. Arch Surg 63:824–833, 1954.
46. Armstrong TJ: Ergonomics and cumulative trauma disorders. Hand Clin 2:553, 1986.
47. Goldstein SA, Armstrong TJ, Chaffin DB: Analysis of cummulative strain in tendons and tendon sheaths. J Biomech 20:1, 1987.
48. Manske PR, Ogata K, Lesker PA: Nutrient pathways to extensor tendons of primates. J Hand Surg (Br) 10B:8, 1985.
49. Runge F: Zur Genese und Behandlung des Schreibekrampfes. Ber Klin Wochenschr 10:245, 1873.
50. Allender E: Prevalence, incidence and remission rates of some common rheumatic diseases or syndromes. Scand J Rheumatol 3:145, 1974.
51. Bernhang AM: The many causes of tennis elbow. NY State J Med 79:1363, 1979.
52. Hohmann G: Ueber den Tennisellenbogen. Verh Dtsch Orthop Ges 21:349, 1927.
53. Garden RS: Tennis elbow. J Bone Joint Surg (Br) 43B:100, 1961.
54. Roles NC, Maudsley RH: Radial tunnel syndrome. J Bone Joint Surg (Br) 54B:499, 1972.
55. Van Rossum J, Buruma OJS, Kamphuisen HAC, Onylee GJ: Tennis elbow—a radial tunnel syndrome? J Bone Joint Surg (Br) 60B:197, 1978.
56. Beenisch J, Wilhelm K: Die Epicondylitis humeri lateralis: Aetiopathogenesese und Behandlungserfolg. Fortschr Med 103:417, 1985.

57. Wilhelm A: Die Eingriffe zur Schmerzausschaltung durch Denervation. In: Wachs-muth W, Wilhelm A (eds): Allgemeine und Spezielle Chirurgische Operationslehre. Dritter Teil: Die Operationen an der Hand. Springer-Verlag, Berlin, 1972, pp 266–269.
58. Schneider H, Corradini V: Aufbrauch-veranderungen in sehr beanspruchten Schnen der oberen Extremitaet und ihre klinische Bedeutung. Z Orthop 84:296–352, 1954.
59. Price R, Sinclair H, Heinrich I, et al.: Local injection treatment of tennis elbow–hydrocortisone, triamcinolone, and lignocaine compared. Br J Rheumatol 30:39–44, 1991.
60. Kivi P: The etiology and conservative treatment of humeral epicondylitis. Scand J Rehabil Med 15:37–41, 1982.
61. Brattberg G: Acupuncture therapy for tennis elbow. Pain 16:285–288, 1983.
62. Gillman H: Tennis elbow (lateral epicondylitis). Common hand problems. Szabo RM (ed): Orthop Clin North Am 23:75–82, 1992.
63. Cummings GS, Tillman LJ: Remodeling of dense connective tissue in normal adult tissues. In Currier DP, Nelson RM (eds): Dynamics of Human Biological Tissues. FA Davis, Philadelphia, 1992, pp 45–73.
64. Enwemeka CS, Spielholz NI: Modulation of tendon growth and regeneration by electrical fields and currents. In Currier DP, Nelson RM (eds): Dynamics in Human Biological Tissues. FA Davis, Philadelphia, 1993, pp 231–254.

CHAPTER 5

Fractures and Dislocations of the Wrist, Hand, and Fingers

In all hand and wrist fractures, knowledge of normal anatomy of the part is necessary to insure proper management. The metacarpals participate in three arches: the proximal, the distal transverse, and the longitudinal. The proximal carpal arch, formed by the carpal bones, has already been discussed (see Chapter 1). The distal transverse arch comprises the distal portions of the metacarpal heads, and the longitudinal arch can be seen from the side (Fig. 5–1).[1] The index and middle metacarpals have little mobility, whereas the other metacarpals are more mobile (see Chapter 1).

The carpometacarpal joints are relatively immobile due to the congruity of their articulations, which are reinforced by stout dorsal and palmar ligaments. The metacarpolphalangeal joints gain stability through their collateral ligaments and their volar plates.

There is no motion at the index and middle fingers, whereas the ring finger moves 15° and the little finger 25°. The thumb flexes 50°, abducts 40°, and rotates 17°. The interosseus muscles flex the metacarpolphalangeal (MP) joints, extend the interphalangeal (IP) joints, and abduct or adduct the digits. These muscles are the deforming forces in metacarpal neck and shaft fractures, with the deformity being of the apex dorsal angulation.

PRINCIPLES OF TREATMENT

Fractures and dislocations of the fingers have frequently been ignored or cursorily treated, with resultant severe disability. Loss of

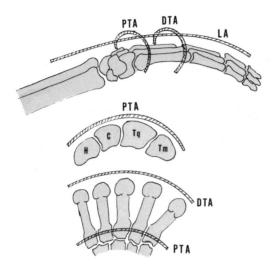

Figure 5–1. Three arches of the metacarpals. The three arches of the metacarpals are the proximal transverse arch (PTA) formed by the carpal bones: the trapezium (Tm), trapezoid (Tq), capitiate (C), and the hamate (H). The distal transverse arch (DTA) formed by the heads of the five metacarpals and the longitudinal arch (LA) by all the bones of the hand viewed laterally.

finger function interferes markedly with use of the upper extremity and is a cause of significant vocational attrition.

The following principles in the care of injured phalanges and interphalangeal joints must not be violated:

1. Immobilization must be instituted to relieve pain and permit primary healing. Too early, or inappropriate, active or passive motion may result in more pain and contracture. Usually immobilization must be maintained for at least 10 to 14 days.
2. Immobilization must be maintained in degrees of physiologic flexion listed in Fig. 5–2. No fracture must be immobilized with extension of all three joints.
3. All digits that do not require immobilization must be actively, not passively, mobilized.

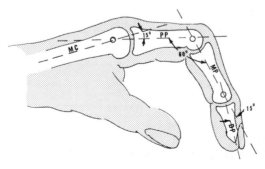

Figure 5–2. Position of physiological immobilization in the treatment of fractures. Immobilization of the joints of the fingers in treatment of fractures is best done with 15° of the metacarpophalangeal joint (MC) – (PP), 60° at the proximal interphalangeal joint (PP) – (MP), and 15° at the distal joints (MP) – (DP).

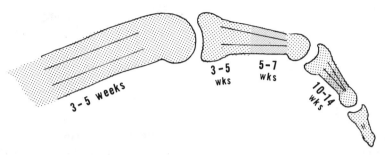

Figure 5–3. Fracture healing time. Bone that is more vascular and canellous (proximal bones) heals more rapidly that denser bone (distal). It is not necessary to immobilize fractures for these length of time. (Modified from Moberg E: Emergency Surgery of the Hand. Livingstone, London, 1967.)

4. The uninvolved digits of the hand, wrist, elbow, and shoulder must be actively placed through their normal range of motion, with emphasis upon frequent elevation of the hand above heart level.

The duration of immobilization is "not equated with the time of healing: it is shorter than this time factor."[2] (see Fig. 5–3.) Active range-of-motion exercises must be started before x-ray films show evidence of healing, usually within 1 to 2 weeks.

METACARPAL FRACTURES AND DISLOCATIONS

Metacarpal Head Fractures

These fractures are usually the result of direct trauma and ordinarily involve the border digits—the index and little fingers. The more common fracture is an avulsion of the collateral ligament, with intra-articular fractures being less common but more disabling, as the fragments are difficult to reduce. A residual displacement of 1 to 2 mm after healing predisposes to poor results.[3]

Treatment protocols for these fractures are rare, as there are few long-term follow-up reports. Nonoperative treatment is indicated if the fracture is stable to active stress, and consists of immobilization for 2 to 3 weeks with 30° of wrist extension, MP joints at 90° flexion, and the IP joints fully extended.

Open reduction is indicated if there is instability with stress, a loss of articular integrity, and more than 20-percent involvement of the articular surface.[4] Reduction and immobilization are accomplished by use of K-wires (Kirschner wires) or screws, followed by active and passive movement.[5]

Metacarpal Neck Fractures

These fracture are the more common hand fractures and occur from a direct blow to the closed fist. Resultant angulation or rotational deformity may occur (Fig. 5–4). Closed reduction can be accomplished with the PIP and MP joints flexed to 90°.[6] (See Fig. 5–5.)

Fractures of the fifth metacarpal neck must be mobilized immediately, regardless of the incurred angulation, to ensure good functional recovery.[7]

Other metacarpal neck fractures may need internal fixation if there is rotational malalignment and adequate fixation cannot be maintained. Percutaneous pinning appears to be the technique of choice,[8] with open reduction rarely indicated except in irreducible fractures.

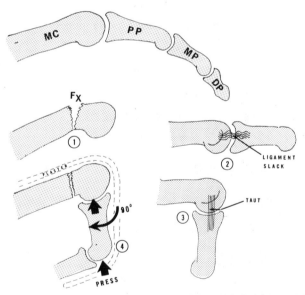

Figure 5–4. Metacarpal neck fractures. (1) The usual deformity of the distal fragment. (2) As the lateral ligaments are slack in the extended position the fracture 'cannot' be reduced with the fingers in this position. (3) In the flexed finger position the lateral ligaments become taut and the metacarpophalangeal joint is immobile thus the proximal phalanx can be used to reduce the metacarpal neck fracture by exertion of the forces (dark arrows) (see Fig. 5–5.) A dorsal splint is then applied for 3 weeks.

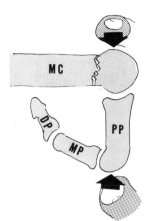

Figure 5–5. Closed reduction of fracture of the metacarpal neck. With the flexed metacarpal (MC) phalangeal (PP) joint flexed to 90°, which makes taut the lateral ligaments, the fingers of the physician (dark arrows) can reduce the carpal neck fracture.

Inadequate reduction may result in loss of the dorsal contour of the MP joint and cause a prominence of the head in the palm;[9] the result is a painful grasp and/or hyperextension of the MP joint.

In summary, treatment of fractures of the metacarpal neck requires reduction for less than 3 weeks immobilization if there is less than 10° to 15° of palmar angulation in the index and middle fingers, 35° in the ring metacarpal, or 45° in the little metacarpal. If these limitations are exceeded, closed reduction is indicated, followed by splint or cast immobilization for 3 to 4 weeks while keeping the distal phalanges free.

Metacarpal Shaft Fractures

These fractures present a different problem of management than do the fractures of the neck, as angular deformity is less acceptable and fractures tend to be oblique, transverse, or spiral. Reduction is acceptable only if there is less than 10° angulation of the index and middle metacarpals, 20° angulation of the ring metacarpal, and 3 mm of shortening and rotation.[10] Most fractures can be reduced and immobilized for 4 to 6 weeks in an external splint that includes the wrist and entire metacarpal shaft but not the MP joint. The mold must cover the dorsum of the fracture site and the palmar aspect of the metacarpal head. After 4 weeks these fractures, although showing no evidence of union on x-rays,[11] are sufficiently stable to permit slight active motion.

Fractures at the base of a metacarpal are usually innocuous and merely need reduction by manual manipulation (Fig. 5–6) and dorsal splinting, with simultaneous active exercises of the fingers and thumb. If the fragments cannot be held together, open reduction and immobilization with an intramedullary Kirschner wire may be needed.

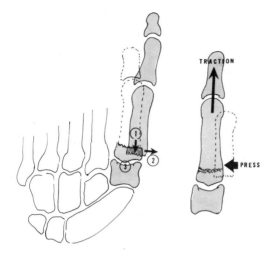

Figure 5–6. Simple impacted fracture of base of thumb metacarpal. Fracture of the base of the thumb metacarpal with impaction (1) and lateral displacement (2) but no involvement of the joint (3) is treated by reduction done with traction and simultaneous pressure against the distal fragment. The fracture is then casted.

Treatment must never immobilize any of the digits or the metacarpal joints. Frequent active exercises to maintain full range of motion with the hand elevated must be instituted and supervised.

Complications of this type of fracture include joint stiffness, nonunion, malunion, and tendon rupture, so that these fractures must be carefully observed.

Thumb: Metacarpal Shaft Fractures, and Metacarpal Fractures and Dislocations

Most fractures involve the proximal quarter of the shaft, with the distal fragment being adducted and supinated. Treatment consists of longitudinal traction (Fig. 5–7), with a well-molded spica splint applied to the thumb for 3 to 4 weeks.[12]

It is important to determine whether the fracture is intra-articular or extra-articular,[13] as the latter are usually stable after reduction, and up to 30° of angulation can be accepted. Intra-articular fractures are usually unstable and require pinning after reduction; they may even require open reduction if joint congruity cannot be achieved. The reduction employs traction, abduction, and pronation of the fragment, with pinning to the trapezium or the second metacarpal.

Rolando described a Bennett fracture with the addition of a palmar fragment of the metacarpal.[14] Such fractures are relatively uncommon but demand open reduction and pinning.

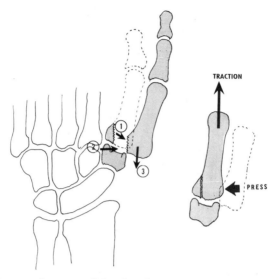

Figure 5-7. Bennett fracture of the thumb metacarpal. This is a fracture of the base of the thumb metacarpal with lateral displacement. 1 shows fracture through the base; 2 shows proximal dislocation; 3, the dislocation is aggravated by the pull of the flexor and extensor tendons. This fracture is reduced by traction with simultaneous pressure against the distal fragment. Prognosis is guarded because of residual instability and ultimate degenerative arthritis.

Fractures and Dislocations of the First to Fifth Metacarpals

Dislocations and fracture dislocations of the index to the fifth metacarpals are uncommon, but as they occur usually in violent accidents that involve other fractures, they are frequently missed.[15] As the metacarpals are located in a side-by-side position, a fracture dislocation of one should arouse suspicion of an adjacent injury.[16]

Medial (ulnar direction) dislocations of the fifth metacarpal usually can be simply reduced, but preventing repeat dislocation may be more difficult and may require skeletal fixation. Lateral (radial direction) dislocation usually requires open reduction. Persistent subluxation and incongruity may lead to pain and grip weakness.[17]

Dislocations may disrupt the normal transverse and longitudinal arches, and this disruption may impair the grip strength and upset the intrinsic-extrinsic extensor muscle balance.

Metacarpophalangeal dislocations are less common that PIP dislocations.[18]

METACARPOPHALANGEAL
DISLOCATIONS

Because of the support system of the MP joints, dislocations are significantly less common than PIP dislocations. As stated, the collateral ligaments are slack in extension and taut in flexion, thus creating stability of the extended digits. The volar plate (Fig. 1 – 49) has a thin origin proximal to the metacarpal neck, which becomes thicker distally where it attaches upon the proximal phalanx. These plates are interconnected via the deep transverse intermetacarpal ligaments so as to give additional stability. Volar (palmar) dislocations are rare.[19]

Dorsal dislocations occur from hyperextension injuries and are either simple or complex. In the simple dislocation, the joint may be hyperextended 60° to 90° but the volar plate is not interposed into the joint. These dislocations merely require manual reduction, and splinting with the finger flexed 60°. Complex dislocations tear the volar plate from its proximal site or origin[20] and are more significant, as the plate becomes interposed into the joint (Fig. 5 – 8). A single attempt may be made to reduce the dislocation, but if it fails an open reduction is indicated.[20]

PHALANGEAL FRACTURES

Fractures of proximal phalanges must be repaired to permit normal active interphalangeal joint motion and appropriate tendon glide.[21] There is a precise interdependence upon the length of the dorsum of

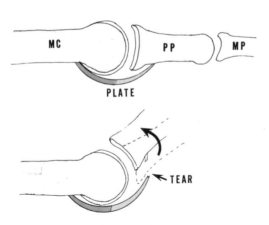

PLATE

TEAR

Figure 5 – 8. Dislocation of the metacarpophalangeal joint. Most fracture dislocations of the metacarpophalangeal joints are hyperextension injuries that either stretch or tear the palmar plate. The proximal plate is thicker and fibrous whereas the distal plate is thin. The distal site is the site of tearing with dorsal subluxation of the proximal phalanx (PP) upon the metacarpal (MC). The middle phalanx (MP) is not involved.

the phalanx and the length of the extensor tendon. The flexor tendons in their fibro-osseous tunnels define the rotational axis of function and thus of deformation after facture. These anatomical inter-relationships determine the appropriate treatment and expected outcome of phalangeal fractures.[22] The intricate mechanisms of finger function demand a precise relationship of extensor and flexor mechanisms, and any disruption of this relationship will impair digital function.[23]

The superficialis and profundus tendons join the transverse and cruciate fibers of their fibro-osseous tunnels, which cover the entire palmar surface of each bone (see Fig. 2–54). Displaced shaft fractures can expose these tendons to the sharp edges of the bone. The extensor mechanism forms the "hood" (see Fig. 1–78) that extends the phalanx. A shaft fracture causing angulation also causes a diminution in the length of the finger and impairment of the extensor mechanism[24] (Fig. 5–9).

Functional loss does not result from fractures of the metacarpals since there is no angulation to cause a dissociation of the extensor-flexor mechanism. Palmar angulation of proximal phalangeal fractures allows ligamentous function, but with secondary flexion contractures and the loss of interphalangeal extension.

A phalangeal fracture that tears the periosteum results in the segments being held together by only the extensor and flexor tendons and their partially torn fibro-osseous tunnel. This flexor remnant forms a "tether" about which the distal segment undergoes rotational displacement (Fig. 5–10). This displacement changes the dynamics of the extensor-flexor mechanisms with resultant palmar angulation and secondary extensor mechanism incompetence due to a change in the length of the phalanx. The "passive" force of the unopposed flexor mechanism expended upon the fracture site compounds the angulation-rotational deformation.

Radiological studies will reveal skeletal alignment and length restoration but not rotational deformation. This rotational malalignment can be clinically ascertained by passively flexing the wrist. This action causes a tenodesis effect upon the PIP joints, and by passive flexion of the wrist and the MP joint, rotation of the distal fragment can be determined.

For the above reasons, closed manual reduction of a proximal phalangeal fracture may realign the length of the shaft without controlling or correcting the rotational angulation. Thus open reduction with Kirschner wire fixation is usually indicated.

Treatment must rely upon the experience and expertise of the hand surgeon as to precise technique. The intent is realignment that ensures unrestricted gliding of the extensor and flexor tendons, with diminution of significant angulation and rotation of the distal fragment.

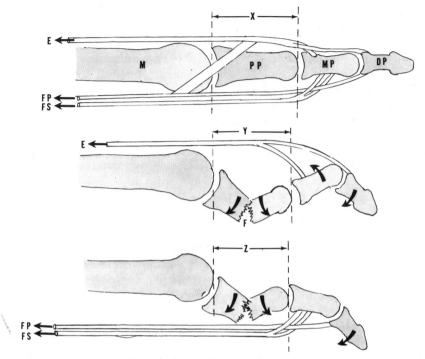

Figure 5–9. Abnormal extensor mechanism from phalangeal fractures. The upper figure depicts the normal attachment of the extensor mechanism (E) and the flexor mechanisms: flexor profundus (FP) and flexor sublimis (FS). Their attachments upon the middle phalanx (MP) and distal phalanx (DP) are shown. X depicts the distance between the proximal and distal margins of the proximal phalanx (PP). The middle illustration shows that a middle phalanx fracture (F) causes palmar bowing with shortening of the length of the phalanx (Y). This changes the functional length of the extensor and flexor mechanisms causing extension of the middle phalanx and flexion of the distal phalanx. The third illustration shows further shortening of the length of the phalanx (Z) from contraction of the flexor mechanism. Failure to correct the length and immobilization of the middle phalanx and maintainence of active motion of the proximal and distal joint range of motion permits contracture of the hand in this position.

Fracture of the middle phalanx tends to bow the finger because of the pull of the flexor digitorum sublimis on the proximal phalanx (Fig. 5–11). Fractures of the proximal portion may angulate dorsally because of the imbalanced extensor mechanism pull (Z in Fig. 5–11).

Rehabilitation of phalangeal fractures must address potential stiffness of the phalanges from pain and swelling. These can cause scarring between the tendon and bony surfaces due to edema and hemorrhage,

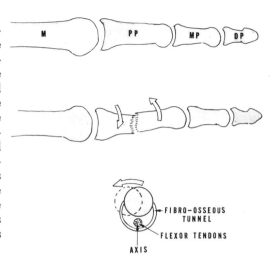

Figure 5-10. Rotational deformity of a fracture of the proximal phalanx. The extensor and flexor tendons of the fingers do not exert their pull in a direct alignment of the finger and a fracture of the middle phalanx often undergoes rotation of the distal fragment upon the proximal fragment (curved arrows in the *middle drawing*). The rotation occurs about the "axis" of the flexor tendons within their fibro-osseous tunnel (*lower drawing*).

albeit on a microscopic scale.[25] To avoid stiffness, the recommended treatment is a splint holding the wrist in slight extension and the fingers in flexion. There should be early active range-of-motion exercises, and the hand should be frequently elevated above heart level. Splints are fully discussed in Chapter 10 and the precise type necessary can be determined from information found there.

Further discussion on dislocations appears in Chapter 6, but dislocation of the thumb is covered here as the thumb metacarpolphalangeal joint is the one most subject to dislocation from hyperextension. The proximal phalanx usually displaces dorsally and the head of the metacarpal may protrude through an associated capsular tear (Fig. 5-12). The capsule and flexor tendons "buttonhole" the head of the metacarpal and maintain the dislocation, with the result that open reduction and capsular repair are necessary.

GAMEKEEPER'S THUMB

Injury to the ulnar collateral ligament and resulting instability of the thumb may be due to pathology of the dorsal aponeurotic insertion of the adductor pollicis.[26] Interest in this condition increased when it became prevalent in skiers.[27]

Two-thirds of the thumb (MCP) diarthrodial ginglimoid joint is metacarpophalangeal coated with a fibrocartilaginous plate, the proximal third of which is very thin (pars flaccida). The ulnar collateral ligament is a 4- to 8-mm band, 12 to 14 mm in length, that inserts upon

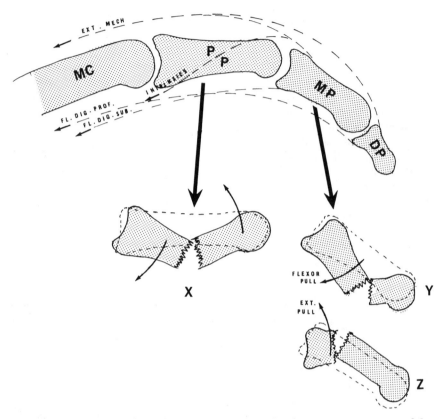

Figure 5-11. Phalangeal fractures, mechanism of deformation. Fractures of the shaft of the proximal phalanx (PP) bow in a palmar direction because of the pull of the intrinsics (lumbricals and interossei) which flex the proximal and extend the distal fragments (X). In fractures of the middle phalanx (MP) at the distal shaft (Y), the proximal fragment flexes because of the pull of the flexor tendons. In a fracture through the proximal shaft (Z), the extensor mechanism acting upon the distal fragment causes dorsal bowing. Regardless of the site or direction of bowing, the treatment consists of traction, reduction, and casting in the flexed position.

the lateral tubercle of the proximal phalanx. The adductor pollicis inserts, via three fila, first into the ulnar sesamoid, then into the lateral tubercle of the proximal phalanx, and finally into a dorsal expansion of the adductor aponeurosis.[28]

The thumb MCP moves predominantly in flexion-extension (10° to 100° and 0° to 90°, respectively), and shows limited rotation.[29] The palmar plate glides during flexion-extension. Passive abduction of 0° to 20° is possible.

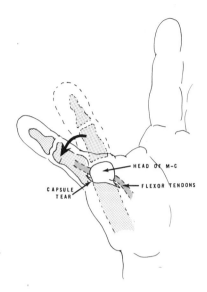

Figure 5–12. Dislocation of metacarpo-phalangeal joint of the thumb. The phalanx displaces backward, tearing the capsule. The head of the metacarpal protrudes through the capsule tear and gets buttonholed in the tear and by the flexor tendon passing behind the head.

Determination of instability is made clinically by weakness in pinch,[30] swelling over the joint, and tenderness over the joint that is aggravated by excessive passive motion.[31,32] Radiological confirmation is possible.[33] Surgical repair is presently recommended.[34]

SCAPHOID FRACTURES

Among the carpal bones, the scaphoid is second only to the distal radius in the frequency of fracture. These fractures occur largely as a result of a fall on the outstretched dorsiflexed hand.

The healing potential and complications leading to nonunion depend on the anatomical structure of the bone. The scaphoid connects the proximal and distal carpal rows, and lies oblique to the longitudinal axis of the carpus on the radial aspect of the wrist. Two-thirds of its surface is covered with cartilage, as it articulates with four adjacent carpal bones and the distal radius (Fig. 5–13).

The volar surface of the scaphoid is concave and nonarticular. The dorsum is convex, with a roughened oblique ridge, upon which attach the distal radial carpal ligaments and along which course the dorsal arterial branches.

The ligaments (Fig. 5–13A) connect the radius with the scaphoid and capitiate (RSCL) and the radius to the scaphoid and lunate bones (RSLL). The V ligaments course from the scaphoid to the capitate and from the capitate to the triquetrum.[35]

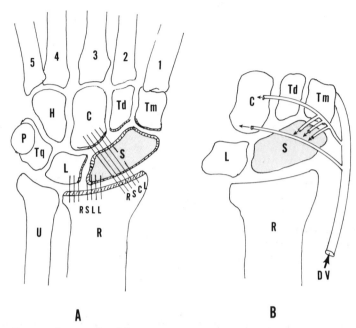

A   B

Figure 5–13. The scaphoid bone. The anatomy is vital in understanding the pathomechanics of fracture healing. (A) The scaphoid bone articulates with five (5) bones: the radius (R) lunate (L), capitate, trapezoid (Td) and trapezium (Tm). The articulations have cartilage (drawn). The ligaments that support the scapoid are sparse: the radio-scapho-lunate ligament (RSLL) and the radio-sca-pho-capitate ligaments (RSCL). The V ligaments (not shown) course from the scaphoid to the capitate from where it courses to the triquetrium. (B) The blood supply to the capitate is primarily from dorsal vessels (DV) and ventral vessels (not shown) from the radial artery. The blood vessels enter the scaphoid bone from the non-articular surfaces: dorsal and volar.

Blood is supplied chiefly by the radial artery, which has volar and dorsal branches. The volar branches supply 20 to 30 percent of the internal vascularization of the distal aspect of the bone.[36,37]

Pathomechanics of Fracture

When a patient falls on the extended arm and dorsiflexed wrist, force is directed through the thenar eminence to the trapezium, and from thence through the scaphoid to the radius. The scaphoid is supported proximally by the radio-scapho-lunate ligaments but has weak distal support. In wrist extension, the scaphoid bone impinges between

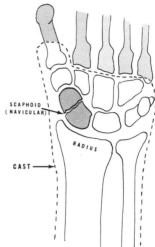

Figure 5–14. Fracture of the carpal scaphoid bone. This fracture is frequently missed on the initial x-ray examination and may require three views to reveal a hairline fracture. Suspicion is aroused by tenderness over the "snuff box," swelling, and painful wrist motion. The fracture should be treated by 6 to 8 weeks of a snug plaster cast that includes the thumb metacarpal and extends to the carpometacarpal joints of the other fingers.

the dorsal lip of the radius and the palmar sling of the radio-scapho-capitate ligament, so that it sustains compressive forces from a fall.

Kinematically the scaphoid normally moves with the proximal carpal row in flexion and extension (see Chapter 1); it flexes when the wrist deviates radially and extends when the wrist deviates in an ulnar direction. The degree of ulnar or radial deviation of the wrist at the time of fall determines where the scaphoid sustains fracture (Fig. 5–14): proximal, dorsal, or at the waist.[38,39] Scaphoid fractures are further classified as (a) tubercle, (b) horizontal oblique, (c) transverse, or (d) vertical oblique (Fig. 5–15). Two-thirds of scaphoid fractures occur in the middle third of the bone and these are equally divided between transverse and oblique fractures.[40]

Clinical Evaluation

The typical history is a fall on the outstretched hand. Clinically there is no wrist deformity other than a swelling on the radial side. Wrist movement is painful and limited, and there is tenderness on palpation of the scaphoid, which can be apprehended in the "snuff box" (Fig. 1–29) between the extensor pollicis longus and extensor pollicis brevis tendons (Fig. 5–16).

Diagnosis may be confirmed by radiographic studies, but multiple views may be "negative" in spite of the presence of a fracture. Hence further studies, either bone scan[41] or tomography,[42] may be needed to

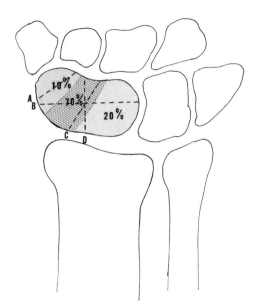

Figure 5–15. Classification of scaphoid fractures. (A) Tubercle; (B) horizontal oblique; (C) transverse; (D) vertical oblique. Based on the blood supply the frequency of occurrences vary from 10% distal, 70% middle, and 20% proximal.

Figure 5–16. Rupture of the extensor pollicis longus. The extensor pollicis longus extends to the distal phalanx along a diagonal course. Its rupture results in loss of extension of the distal digit of the thumb, and some weakness of extension of the proximal joint. The ruptured tendon retracts considerably. End-to-end suture is not feasible, and grafting is required. Rather than extending the laceration, a proximal incision to locate the distal tendon must be made, and the graft is then passed through the canal with a smooth probe.

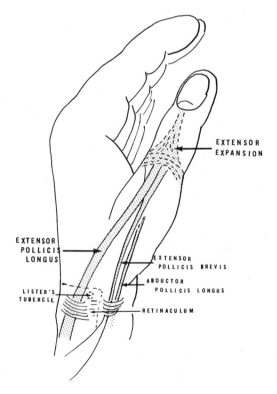

confirm and designate the site and classification of fracture. In the presence of a probable fracture with negative x-rays, appropriate treatment should be instituted,[41] with further studies performed in 2 weeks. Scaphoid fractures may also occur in conjunction with fractures of the distal radius or fractures of the elbow,[43] and should always be evaluated.

Treatment

The anatomy of the fracture and the amount of displacement or angulation determines the type of treatment. Almost all distal pole and tubercle fractures can be treated with a simple, short arm cast immobilization that includes the thumb.[40] Transverse fractures of the waist without displacement can also be managed by short cast immobilization; however, such fractures, even though undisplaced, may be unstable and can be treated to advantage by casting from below the elbow with incorporation of the thumb. When a fracture is truly unstable, open reduction and internal fixation is indicated.

Stable undisplaced fractures rarely become nonunions and typically heal in 6 to 12 weeks. Again, it must be remembered that routine x-rays may not show union; thus tomograms may be indicated. All patients sustaining a carpal fracture should be revaluated 6 to 12 months after cessation of treatment.

A malunion is nearly always symptomatic.[44] Such cases must be recognized early and treated promptly by techniques of open reduction or percutaneous pinning that are beyond the scope of this text. After 6 months with no evidence of healing, appropriate casting is still worth consideration, and healing may be enhanced by electrical stimulation.[45]

When a scaphoid fracture fails to heal, the natural history is development of radioscaphoid then capitolunate post-traumatic arthritis.[46] Surgical salvage may need to be considered, including carpectomy.[47] All these complications and possible malunions indicate the need for early diagnosis, correct classification, and appropriate treatment to obviate the possibility of nonunion or malunion.

DISTAL RADIAL FRACTURES

The fundamental principle underlying treatment of the distal radial fracture is restoration of the articular congruity of the distal joints for functional restoration of painless motion of the wrist and fingers. Essentially this implies the restoration of normal anatomical relationships.

The most common wrist fracture is the Colles' fracture, in which a fracture through the distal radius causes the distal fragment to be dis-

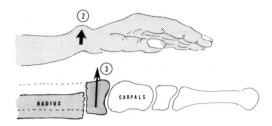

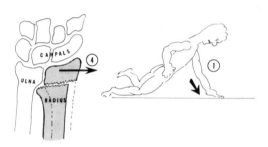

Figure 5–17. Colles' fracture. (1) Fracture usually occurs from a fall upon the outstretched hand. (2) The typical "dinner-fork" or "silver-fork" deformity is noted. (3) The distal fragment is displaced backward (dorsally) and (4) outward (radially).

placed radially or dorsally. The resultant deformity is termed "silver fork" or "dinner forked" (Fig. 5–17). This fracture usually occurs from a fall on the outstretched hand with the wrist in 40° to 90° of dorsiflexion.[48] Besides the direct result (malalignment of the radial-carpal articulation), the sequelae of these fractures, including nerve damage, are potentially ominous.

The magnitude and direction of the force causing the fracture and the condition of the bone will determine the injury pattern. With the wrist in extension at the time of the fall, there are compressive forces upon the dorsal aspects of the radius and traction upon the palmar tissues. The adjacent lunate can exert a compressive force upon the distal radius with resultant compressive fracture of the lunate, the so-called "die punch feature." The scaphoid can also undergo a depression fracture. When there is a fracture of the ulnar styloid this is an avulsion fracture from the tensile forces transmitted through the fibrocartilaginous complex (see Fig. 1–14).

There are numerous classifications of radial fractures[49,50] with the following relating to all aspects:

Type I: Extra-articular radial fracture.

Type II: Extra-articular radial fracture with an ulnar styloid fracture.

Type III: Intra-articular fracture of the radiocarpal joint.

Type IV: Intra-articular fracture of the radius with an ulnar styloid fracture.

Type V: Fracture of the radioulnar joint.

Type VI: Fracture of the radioulnar joint with an ulnar styloid fracture.

Type VII: Intra-articular fracture involving both radiocarpal and radioulnar joints.

Type VIII: Intra-articular fracture involving both radiocarpal and radioulnar joints with an ulnar styloid fracture.

Treatment

Treatment obviously is dictated by the severity and the inclusion of any and/or all components of the fracture(s). Evaluation of the immediate status of the adjacent nerve(s) is mandated. This involves predominantly the median nerve (Fig. 1–22), which can be impaired due to compression by edema within the carpal tunnel. This is considered an acute carpal tunnel median nerve compression syndrome (see Chapter 2). Along with the clinical manifestations of median nerve compression, lateral radiograms can ascertain the degree of shortening and angulation, as well as soft tissue swelling. Immediate decompression is mandated.[51]

Carpal tunnel pressures have been measured in varying degrees of wrist positions with Colles' fractures (Fig. 5–18)[51] which plays a role in the slab/cast positions during treatment.

Stable Fractures. Minimally displaced and noncomminuted fractures (types I and II) can be treated with closed reduction (Fig. 5–19) and dorsal-palmar, above-the-elbow plaster slabs; the wrist is positioned in 10° to 20° degrees flexion and 15° ulnar deviation.

Within these slabs finger active range of motion is encouraged. When swelling has subsided, the slabs are replaced by a cast that imobilizes the elbow. The cast is employed for 6 weeks, followed by a palmar wrist splint for an additional 2 weeks when gentle wrist flexibility exercises are begun.

Unstable Fractures. When distal radial fractures fail to heal, they essentially become unstable and symptomatic. Treatment here demands clarification of the precise extent of the fractures (Fig. 5–20) so that the percutaneous pinning includes all aspects of the fractures involved. Whether pinning, plaster, or both are indicated depends on the experience of the orthopedic surgeon and is beyond the scope of this text.

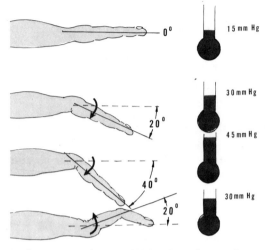

Figure 5–18. Pressure variants within the carpal tunnel related to wrist position. Dependent upon the position of the wrist the pressure within the carpal tunnel varies. A pressure of 40 mm Hg threatens the viability of the median nerve. The least pressure is with the wrist in the neutral position (0°). Colles' fractures change to position of the wrist as does edema following trauma. The position of splinting also demands consideration of this fact. (Modified from Gelberman RH, Szabo RM, Mortensen WW: Carpal tunnel pressures and wrist position in patients with Colles fractures. Trauma 24: 748, 1984.)

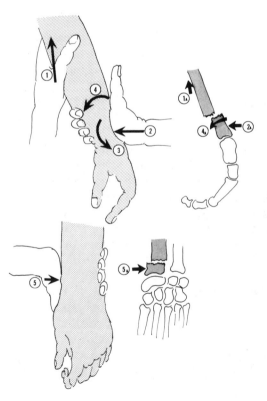

Figure 5–19. Reduction of Colles' fracture. (1) Traction is applied in a proximal direction by immobilizing the forearm with one hand. (2) The thenar eminence of the manipulating hand presses the radial fragment posteriorly causing (3) ulnar deviation. As the fragment slips into place, the forearm is (4) pronated. (5) A new grip is then taken and the fragment is pushed inward (ulnarly). The forearm is then casted in a carefully molded plaster.

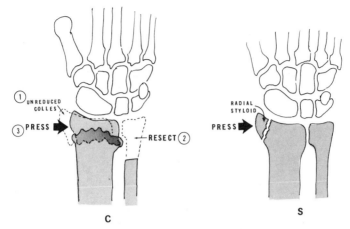

Figure 5-20. Treatment of an unreduced Colles' fracture; treatment of radial styloid fracture. (C) After 6 to 8 weeks, the unreduced Colles' fracture cannot be reduced simply. The ulna can be resected, then the radial fragment can be manipulated into position. (S) If the styloid process of the radius can be reduced by direct pressure, it should be casted for 4 weeks.

The use of distraction also must be considered[52]; this may be necessary so as to not place the entensor tendons under undue tension, which can ultimately cause a "claw hand," that is, extension of the metacarpolphalangeal joints, with flexion of the proximal interphalangeal joints contracted in the flexed position.[53]

Involvement of the scaphoid bone as a sequelae of a fractured distal radius has been discussed.

REFERENCES

1. American Society for Surgery of the Hand: Regional Review Course in Hand Surgery Syllabus, ed 10. ASSH, Aurora, Colo., 1990, pp 9-12.
2. Moberg E: Emergency Surgery of the Hand. E & S Livingstone, London, 1967.
3. Hastings H, Carroll C: Treatment of closed articular fractures of the metacarpalphalangeal and proximal interphalangeal joints. Hand Clin 4:503-527, 1988.
4. McElfresh E, Dobyns J: Intra-articular metacarpal head fractures. J Hand Surg (Br) 8:383-393, 1983.
5. Rayhack J, Bottke C: Intraosseous compression wiring of displaced articular condylar fractures. J Hand Surg (Am) 15A:370-373, 1990.
6. American Society for Surgery of the Hand: Regional Review Course in Hand Surgery Syllabus, ed 10. ASSH, Aurora, Colo., 1990, pp 8-9.
7. Ford D, Ali M, Steel W: Fractures of the fifth metacarpal neck: is reduction or immobilization necessary? J Hand Surg (Br) 14B:165-167, 1989.

8. Melone C: Rigid fixation of phalangeal and metacarpal fractures. Orthop Clin North Am 17:421–435, 1986.
9. Zemel N, Stark H: Problem fractures and dislocations of the hand. Am Assoc Orthop Surg Instructional Course Lectures, 1990, pp 235–249.
10. O'Brien ET: Fractures of the metacarpals and phalanges. In Green DP (ed): Operative Hand Surgery, ed 2. New York, Churchill Livingstone, 1988, pp 709–775.
11. Bora FW, Didizian NH: The treatment of injuries to the metacarpal joint of the little finger. J Bone Joint Surg (Am) 56A:1459–1463, 1974.
12. Pellegrini V: Fractures at the base of the thumb. Hand Clin 4:87–103, 1988.
13. Bennett E: The classic: on fracture of the metacarpal bone of the thumb. Clin Orthop 220:3–6, 1987.
14. Breen TF, Gelberman RH, Jupiter JB: Intra-articular fractures of the basilar joint of the thumb. Hand Clin 4:491–501, 1988.
15. Marck K, Klasen H: Fracture-dislocation of the hamatometacarpal joint: a case report. J Hand Surg (Am) 11A:128–130, 1986.
16. Cain J, Shepler T, Wilson M: Hematometacarpal fracture-dislocation: classification and treatment. J Hand Surg (Am) 12A:762–767, 1987.
17. Peterson P, Sacks S: Fracture-dislocation of the base of the fifth metacarpal associated with injury to the deep motor branch of the ulnar nerve: a case report. J Hand Surg (Am) 11A:525–528, 1986.
18. Hubbard L: Metacarpophalangeal dislocations. Hand Clin 4:38–44, 1988.
19. Hastings H, Carroll C: Treatment of closed articular fractures of the metacarpophalangeal and proximal interphalangeal joints. Hand Clin 4:503–527, 1988.
20. Green D, Terry G: Complex dislocations of the metacarpophalangeal joint. J Bone Joint Surg (Am) 55A:1480–1486, 1973.
21. Widgerow AD, Edinburg M, Biddulph SL: An analysis of proximal phalangeal fractures. J Hand Surg (Am) 12A:134–139, 1987.
22. Strickland JW, Steichen JB, Kleinman WB, et al.: Factors influencing digital performance after phalangeal fracture. In Strickland JW, Steichen JB (eds): Difficult Problems in Hand Surgery. CV Mosby, St. Louis, 1982, pp 126–139.
23. Agee J: Treatment principles for proximal and middle phalangeal fracture. Common hand problems. Orthop Clin North Am 23:35–40, 1992.
24. Jones WW: Biomechanics of small bone fixation. Clin Orthop 214:11–18, 1987.
25. Brand PW: Postoperative stiffness and adhesions. In: Clinical Mechanics of the Hand. CV Mosby, St. Louis, 1985, pp 113–126.
26. Mondray F: Beitrag zur Operativen Behandlung des Wackelddaumens. Zentralbl Chir 67:1532–1535, 1940.
27. Gerber C, Senn E, Matter P: Skier's thumb, surgical treatment of recent injuries to the ulnar collateral ligament of the thumb's metacarpophalangeal joint. Am J Sports Med 9:171–177, 1981.
28. Coonrad RW, Goldner JL: A study of the pathological findings and treatment in soft tissue injury of the thumb metacarpophalangeal joint. J Bone Joint Surg 59A:439–451, 1968.
29. Frank WE, Dobyns J: Surgical pathology of collateral ligamentous injuries of the thumb. Clin Orthop 83:102–114, 1972.
30. Watson-Jones R: Fractures and Joint Injuries, ed 3. E & S Livingston, Edinburgh, 1943, p 587.
31. Abrahamsson S, Soillerman C, Lundborg G et al.: Diagnosis of displaced collateral ligament of the metacarpophalangeal joint of the thumb. J Hand Surg (Am) 15A:457–460, 1990.
32. Alldred AJ: Rupture of the collateral ligament of the metacarpophalangeal joint of the thumb. J Bone Joint Surg (Am) 37B:443–445, 1955.

33. Bowers WH, Hurst LC: Gamekeeper's thumb: evaluation by arthrography and stress roentgenography. J Bone Joint Surg (Am) 59A:519–524, 1977.
34. Newland GC: Gamekeeper's thumb. Common hand problems. Orthop Clin North Am 23:41–48, 1992.
35. Spinner M (ed): Kaplan's Functional and Surgical Anatomy of the Hand, ed 3. JB Lippincott, Philadelphia, 1984.
36. Taleisneck J, Kelly PJ: The extraosseous and intraosseous blood supply of the scaphoid bone. J Bone Joint Surg (Am) 48A:1125–1137, 1966.
37. Gelberman RH, Menon J: The vascularity of the scaphoid bone. J Hand Surg (Am) 5:508–513, 1980.
38. Weber E, Chao EY: An experimental approach to the mechanism of scaphoid fractures. J Hand Surg (Am) 2:142–148, 1978.
39. Weber ER: Biomechanical implications of scaphoid wrist fractures. Clin Orthop 149:83–89, 1980.
40. Taleisnik J: Fractures of the carpal bones. In Green DP (ed): Operative Hand Surgery, Vol 2, ed 2. Churchill Livingstone, New York, 1988, p 813.
41. DaCruz DJ, Bodiwala GG, Finlay DBL: The suspected fracture of the scaphoid: a rational approach to diagnosis. Injury 19:149, 1988.
42. Linscheid RL, Dobyns JH, Younge DK: Transpiral tomography in the evaluation of wrist injury. Bull Hosp Jt Dis Orthop Inst 44:297, 1984.
43. Funk DA, Wood MB: Concurrent fractures of the ipsilateral scaphoid and radial head: report of four cases. J Bone Joint Surg 70A:134, 1988.
44. Lindstrom G, Nystrom A: Incidence of post-traumatic arthrosis after primary healing of scaphoid fractures: a clinical and radiological study. J Hand Surg (Br) 15B:11, 1990.
45. Frykman GK, Taleisnik J, Peters G, et al.: Treatment of nonunited scaphoid fractures by pulsed electromagnetic field and cast. J Hand Surg (Am) 11A:344, 1986.
46. Calandra JJ, Goldner RD, Hardaker WT: Scaphoid Fractures: assessment and Treatment (review). Orthopedics 15:931–937, 1992.
47. Amadio PC: Scaphoid fractures. Common hand problems. Orthop Clin North Am 23:7–17, 1992.
48. Frykman G: Fracture of the distal radius including sequelae: shoulder-hand-finger syndrome, disturbances of the distal radio-ulnar joint and impairment of nerve function. A clinical and experimental study. Acta Orthop Scand (Suppl) 108:3, 1967.
49. Gartland JJ, Werley CW: Evaluation of healed Colles' fractures. J Bone Joint Surg (Am) 33A:895–907, 1951.
50. Older TM, Stabler EV, Casselbaum WH: Colles' fracture: evaluation and selection of treatment. J Trauma 5:469–576, 1965.
51. Gelberman RH, Szabo RM, Mortensen WW: Carpal tunnel pressure and wrist position in patients with Colles' fractures. J Trauma 24:747–749, 1984.
52. Seitz WH, Froimson AI, Brooks DB, et al.: Biomechanical analysis of pin placement and pin size for external fixation of distal radius fractures. Clin Orthop 251:207–212, 1990.
53. Weber SC, Szabo RM: Severely comminuted distal radial fracture as an unsolved problem: complications associated with external fixation and pins and plaster techniques. J Hand Surg (Am) 2:157–165, 1986.

CHAPTER 6
Joints: Injuries and Diseases

The material covered here overlaps the topic of fractures and dislocations discussed in Chapter 5, as included here are dislocations, which are injuries to the soft tissues of the joints. Rheumatoid arthritis is primarily a disease of the soft tissues of joints that involves pain, dysfunction, and ultimate deformity. Both topics are included in this chapter because of the similarities in structural changes, symptoms, and impairment.

SPRAINS

The term "sprain" has its origin in the Old French "espraindre" meaning "to wring," it refers to "trauma to a joint that causes pain and disability depending upon the degree of injury to ligaments."[1] This definition is incomplete, as a sprain is essentially a "subluxation" in which the joint has been moved past its physiologic limits; all the joint tissues, as well as the ligaments, may undergo damage. This includes the capsule, the periarticular tendons, and even the articular cartilagenous tissues. A dislocation is thus a temporary displacement of a bone from its normal position in a joint.

The tissue structures involved in joint sprain are the same as those discussed in Chapter 4 in connection with tendon structures. Tendons, ligaments, and capsules are all composed of dense connective tissue (DCT), of which collagen fibers are an integral part. Collagen tissue can physiologically elongate ("creep") and regain its normal length ("recovery"). The stress-strain curve is the common method of describing the mechanical behavior of tendons, and hence the behavior of collagen fibers[2] in tendons, ligaments, and joint capsules.

Joints respond to external stresses, immobilization, and diseases of the involved tissues. "Strain" has been considered to be a force that exceeds physiologic limits, whereas "sprain" has indicated structural changes in the tissues exposed to more than physiologic strain. Luxation has implied a "dislocation" of a joint in which tissue damage is implied in the act, whereas "subluxation" has implied a reducible partial dislocation that has returned to its original status, albeit with possible tissue damage. Pain occurs when there has been involvement of nociception and nociceptors.[3,4]

As many sprains are momentary subluxations that spontaneously reduce, they often escape detection, both clinically and radiologically, and thus tend to be ignored or minimized. Sprains should be considered as "reduced subluxations" with commensurate soft-tissue injury of capsule, tendons, ligaments, plates, and possibly cartilage.

Immediately after a sprain there usually results swelling of the joint, limited motion (both active and passive), possible discoloration, pain, and tenderness. Radiological changes are absent and the clinical examination may reveal either limited active motion or limited (or excessive) passive joint motion. The limited motion results from inflammation and/or hemorrhage,[5] whereas the excessive motion indicates elongation of the restraining tissues — the capsule, tendons, and/or ligaments.

How the connective tissues respond to external stresses and traumas, and how they recover are important in the implementation of therapeutic efforts.

In connective tissue healing, a sequence of cellular and biological events have been documented,[6] as well as the operation of stimulus-response mechanisms that control its structural reformation. When a tendon is severed, a migration of cells invades the damaged area. Initially, during the first week, 75 percent of the cells are leukocytes; but by the third week 86 percent are macrocytes. These cells are followed by an invasion of newborn "fibroblasts," which are in turn followed by capillary endothelial buds. These latter tissue cells gradually develop into mature fibroblasts and mature blood vessels. Collagen fibers develop from these fibroblasts. Within 4 weeks (experimentally) the active cell population disappears, vascularization diminishes, and the "scar" undergoes reformation from imparted mechanical stresses.[6]

This sequence is stimulated by a chemical, "fibronectin" generated from inflammatory tissue.[7] Fibronectin has not been shown to develop from noninflammatory tissues, so inflammation is needed for this process. Essentially, fibroplasia depends upon inflammation secondary to acute or repetitive trauma.[2]

Stress is a physical stimulus that remodels the alignment and ultimate structure of the collagen fibers, ensuring that there is physiologic creep, and as well as recovery of the normal length and strength of the dense connective tissues of joints that have been injured in subluxation or luxation.

DISLOCATIONS

Sprains of the hand involving the wrist, or fingers imply that excessive forces have been imposed upon a joint.

Dislocation in the Wrist

Dislocations of carpal bones are not extremely common but failure to recognize these dislocations is frequent. The mechanism is usually a fall upon the outstretched extended hand. Radiological diagnosis is frequently misleading, since carpal dislocations are difficult to evaluate in routine radiological studies and injuries are usually ligamentous, with spontaneous realignment.

The most common carpal dislocation is of the perilunate type.[8] (See Fig. 6–1.) The lunate is the bone around which the rest of the carpus dislocates, in either a palmar or a dorsal direction with respect to the lunate. For a significant dislocation to occur, many ligaments must rupture.[9]

If diagnosis is ascertained within the first to third week, treatment is usually closed reduction with casting for 6 to 8 weeks, during which the ligaments heal. If reduction cannot be maintained by casting, percutaneous pinning may be necessary. Gross instability due to severe ligamentous damage may require open reduction and ligamentous repair.[10]

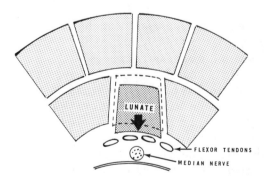

Figure 6–1. Dislocation of the lunate carpal bone. Except for the lunate, all the carpal bones dislocate dorsally because of their shape. From a fall upon the dorsiflexed hand, the lunate dislocates in a palmar direction, causing swelling on the volar surface of the wrist and compression of the flexor tendons of the fingers and median nerve.

Management of dislocations of the wrist must follow the principles of connective tissue healing. Initially edema must be addressed by elevation of the part and active exercises of all distal and proximal joints of the hand; pain should be the guide as to the intensity and force of these active exercises. A static wrist support between exercise periods is permitted for comfort but must not be excessively prolonged. *The goal of treatment is the regaining of normal range of motion and strength.*

The extent of healing of the ligaments depends on manual examination of the stability of the carpus.[11] Passive motion of the wrist may require dynamic splints and active assisted exercises from a therapist.[12] Strengthening exercises must include all the muscles that cross the wrist. Therapeutic putty and "hand helper" exercises are indicated.

Complications. The near presence of the median nerve and the flexor tendons of the fingers means that these must be carefully evaluated (see Fig. 6–1). Persistent pain and stiffness may indicate a partial wrist fusion and/or post-traumatic arthritis, both of which require additional studies, with or without surgical intervention.[5]

Dislocations of the Fingers

The most frequently encountered acute dislocation is dorsal displacement at the proximal interphalangeal joint (PIP), usually from a longitudinal force directed at the tip of the extended finger. Dislocation of this joint implied damage to the supporting structures: the volar plate, and the ulnar and radial collateral ligaments (Fig. 6–2).

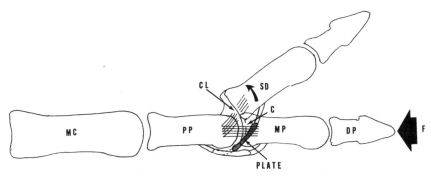

Figure 6–2. Dorsal dislocation of the PIP joint. The longitudinal force (F) expended upon the distal phalanx (DP) of the extended finger causes a hyperextension subluxation (S.D. direction of subluxation) of the articulation of the proximal phalanx (PP) and the middle phalanx (MP). The plate is torn as are the collateral ligaments (CL) and the capsule (C).

Determination of the degree of ligamentous disruption can be ascertained by clinical manual evaluation, in which joint movement and "joint play" are determined (see Fig. 1–16). Ascertaining which soft tissue is damaged and to what degree determines the proper therapeutic approach.

Interphalangeal and metacarpophalangeal dislocations are usually hyperextension injuries, which can be reduced by traction (Fig. 6–3). Most dorsal dislocations are stable following reduction, even those in which there are bony fragments, as long as these involve less than 20 percent of the articular surface.[13]

Initial treatment after reduction demands attention to removal of the edema and immobilization of the PIP joint in 25° to 45° of flexion. The exact degree of flexion depends upon the stability of the joint.[14]

Within 7 to 10 days, when pain and edema has subsided, active motion should be initiated to prevent adhesion of the flexor mechanisms, especially at the volar plate. Both superficialis and profundus exercises should be isolated and emphasized, using electrical stimulation if necessary to insure tendon glide action. Flexion exercises should be initiated within the confines of the digital blocking splint (Fig. 6–4), which prevents extension and allows flexion, both passive and active.

Residual edema, stiffness of the joint, and adhesion of the flexor mechanism is to be avoided. Dynamic traction and gentle "mobilization"[11] of the joint may be required to ensure regaining "joint play."

Within 3 weeks the ligaments, if minimally damaged, should have recovered sufficiently to allow disposal of the dorsal splint that has been

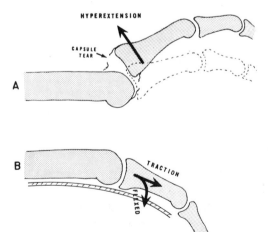

Figure 6–3. Subluxation of metacarpophalangeal joint. (A) The mechanism of subluxation from a hypertension injury in which the capsule may be torn and the head of the metacarpal or the base of the phalanx can herniate. (B) Reduction is by traction and slight flexion, with immobilization in slight flexion for at least three weeks followed by active exercise.

Figure 6-4. Digital dorsal splint. This dorsal blocking splint is molded to ensure 20° to 45° of flexion (curved arrow), allows passive and flexion exercises, and prevents extension until the soft tissues of the PIP joint are ascertained.

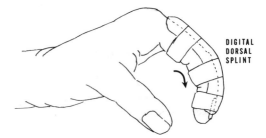

DIGITAL
DORSAL
SPLINT

gradually extended from its original flexed attitude. The digits may be "buddy taped," meaning that the damaged digit is taped to its adjacent digit. The taping allows active and passive range of motion, minimizes excessive extension, and avoids further damage from external sources and inadvertent activities.

The ultimate stage of rehabilitation is the restoration of full range of motion of the PIP joint and regaining full strength of both flexion and extension, usually within 8 weeks. Flexion exercise with therapeutic putty is an excellent modality to mobilize and strengthen the flexor mechanism.

When the dislocation remains unstable, often because of bone fragments (>20% of the articular surface), open reduction is indicated,[14] and the palmar plate is advanced by insertion of a pull-out wire (Fig. 6-5).

The major concern regarding rehabilitation of an extension dislocation is residual swelling and joint stiffness. These result from capsular thickening, as well as fibrosus of the collateral ligaments and adhesions of the flexor mechanism.[15] Pain may enhance and promote this flexion contracture by minimizing therapeutic goals, or treatment may be inadequate and inappropriate.

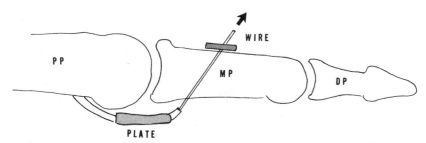

WIRE

PP

MP

DP

PLATE

Figure 6-5. Open reduction of PPP unstable dislocation. The palmar plate is reduced and reattached by a traction wire.

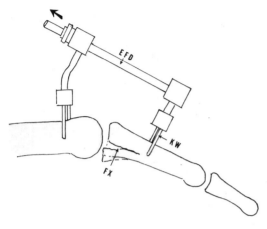

Figure 6–6. External fixation reduction of PIP fracture. A comminuted fracture, with or without subluxation (FX) is reduceable with an external fixation device system (EFD) applying traction (arrow) and utilizing Kirchner wires (KW).

Comminuted intra-articular proximal interphalangeal (PIP) joint fractures, with or without subluxation, are among the most difficult problems in hand surgery. Closed reduction with splinting is simple but often ineffectual in producing or maintaining adequate reduction. Open reduction with internal fixation may restore anatomical alignment but is technically demanding and often results in post-operative stiffness and loss of motion due to periarticular fibrosis.

The recommended procedure is reduction with external fixation (mini Hoffman external fixation system Fig. 6–6) applied under local anesthetic in an operating room.[16] The device is maintained for 3 weeks, after which active range-of-motion exercises are begun.

Salvage procedures may be needed to assure proper digital function. These include arthrodesis or implant arthroplasty, the techniques of which are beyond the scope of this text.

Metacarpophalangeal Dislocation of the Thumb

The metacarpophalangeal thumb joint is the digit most subject to dislocation from external forces. The proximal phalanx usually displaces dorsally and the head of the metacarpal may protrude through the associated caspular tear. As mentioned previously (Chapter 5) the capsule and the flexor tendons actually "buttonhole" the metacarpal head and maintain the dislocation (Fig. 6–7). Open reduction and repair of the capsule are usually necessary.

The fifth carpometacarpal joint is also a saddle joint, resembling that the thumb, and is also frequently subjected to dislocating forces.

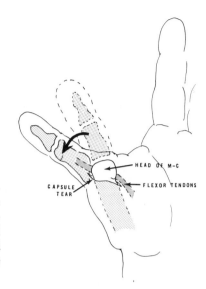

Figure 6-7. Dislocation of metacarpophalangeal joint of the thumb. The phalanx displaces backwards, tearing the capsule. The head of the metacarpal protrudes through the capsule tear and gets buttonholed in the tear and by the flexor tendon passing behind the head.

Open reduction is also often required, along with wire insertion to maintain the reduction. Residual degenerative articular changes often result in painful limitation of motion and the lack of a good grip action.

JOINT STRUCTURE

Extremity joints are diarthrodial (synovial) permitting movement over a wide range of motion. Joints are joined together by a capsule of dense connective tissue compromised of collagen fibers and matrix, ligaments, tendons, and overlying muscles.

The inner surface of the capsules is covered with synovium, a thin layer of cells, under which lies a layer of vascularized connective tissue. The inner layer cells are of two basic types: A, which are active in phagocytosis, and B, which synthesize hyaluronic acid, a lubricant fluid. This hyaluronic fluid is arranged in numerous parallel layers. Pressure at the apex of a joint causes the fluid to move to the wider area of the joint (Fig. 6-8). The synovium is in folds and does not cover the weight-bearing joint cartilage. The inner layer of connective tissue merges with the periosteum of the subchondral bone.

The synovium has a rich network of capillaries, venules, and lymphatics, and is innervated by autonomic (sympathetic) nerves.[14] Some joints contain fibrocartilaginous "discs," which increase the congruity of the joint.[18]

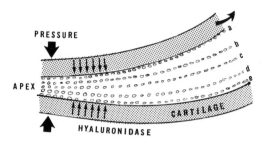

Figure 6-8. Hydrodynamic lubrication. Nonparallel joint surfaces form a wedge-shaped lubricating fluid, some of which stays at the apex. The lubricating fluid moves in layers—a, b, c, d, e,—at the same speed as the articulating bone, but a layer (a-e) adheres to both articular surfaces. A shearing force between layers causes deformation of the fluid. The lubricant is both adhesive and viscous, being coated by hyaluronic acid, which is created by the synovium and cartilage. Even without movement a layer(s) remains between the two opposing joint surfaces.

The cartilage that covers the ends of these bones is composed of type II collagen and proteoglycans, which together provide both form and tensile strength. The proteoglycans comprise 79 percent of the total weight of the cartilage and are constrained by a meshwork of collagen fibers.

Joints are supplied by articular nerves, usually branches of a major adjacent peripheral nerve, and partly by the nerves of adjacent periarticular muscles acting upon that joint. The subsynovial fibrous capsule contains the nerve endings, as well as the blood vessels subserving the joint.

There are four types of nerve endings: type I mechanoreceptors (stretch receptors); type II (resembling Pacinian corpuscles) also mechanoreceptors; type III, resembling Golgi apparatus; and type IV, considered to be nociceptors for pain transmission.

RHEUMATOID ARTHRITIS

Rheumatoid arthritis (RA) is an inflammatory polyarthritis of unknown etiology typically involving peripheral joints in a symmetrical distribution. It is considered to be a systemic autoimmune disease with an unknown causative agent. Women are more commonly afflicted by a ratio of 3:1. Susceptibility to the disease appears to be an inherited trait in a histocompatibility of complex MHC in chromosome 6 involving HLA-DR4.

The disease targets primarily the synovium of joints and tendons, with secondary involvement of the periarticular tissues, muscles, and blood vessels. The hallmark of the disease is the proliferation of synovium, which spreads over the cartilage as pannus.

B cells of the involved synovium take part in an antigen-antibody reaction forming a large molecular weight anti-immuno globulin (IgM class), class otherwise termed "rheumatoid factor" (Fig. 6–9). This factor can be isolated from the serum in a diagnostic procedure.

In the diseased cartilage and synovium, polymorphonuclear white cells attracted by chemotactic factors release phagocytic lysozymes that further damage the cartilage, the synovium of the tendons, and ultimately the subchrondal bone.

The rheumatoid process thus consists of proliferation of the synovial cells, which secrete polymorphonuclear leukocytes; monocytes; and plasma cells, which secrete rheumatoid factor. The lubricant thickens and increases the joint pressure, thus causing mechanical pressure upon the joint tissues. This pressure compounds the damage caused by chemical irritants. The capsule being stretched also thins, and gradually loosens its attachment to the periosteum. The abnormal cells of the synovium migrate across the cartilage in a pannus (Fig. 6–10, A) and also subcortically (Fig. 6–10, B) to gradually damage the cartilage.

The pannus that coats the cartilage inhibits cartilage nutrition, as well as secreting proteolytic enzymes that denude the cartilage. The denuded area becomes the site of fibrocartilagenous tissue formation. The fibrocartilagenous tissue invades the joint space and migrates towards the opposing cartilage that is also undergoing similar cartilage changes. Once there has been a total bridging of the fibrous tissue, ankylosis of the joint occurs.

In the early stages, the thinned capsule allows hypermobility of the joint which increases the potential for further damage due to additional forces on the joint; gradual ankylosis limits motion.

As all these changes are occurring within the joint, the subchondral bone is undergoing atrophy; at the same time, softening and deformation of the bone allow further degenerative changes and possible fractures.

In addition to involvement of the complement system there is also secretion of prostaglandins, leukotrienes, and free oxygen radicals. Prostaglandin PGE_2 is a potent vasodilator and enhances the action of histamine and bradykinin in producing edema and PAIN. The leukotrienes, like prostaglandins, are derived from arachidonic acid and produces smooth muscle contraction. These chemical changes are responsible for the signs and symptoms of rheumatoid arthritic episodes.

Symptoms and Signs

Constitutional symptoms, usually in a young middle-aged woman, are fatigue, weight loss, low-grade fever, and "stiffness" of the hands upon awakening. The hand stiffness may increase and become prolonged, often impairing the usual activities of daily living.

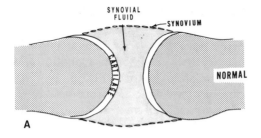

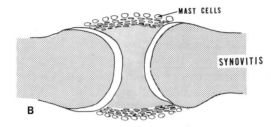

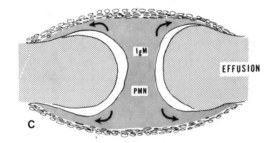

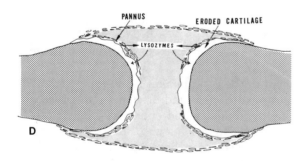

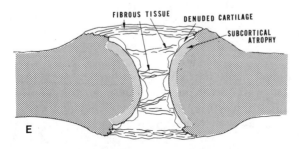

Figure 6–9. Progressive changes of joints in rheumatoid arthritis. *(A)* The normal joint with cartilage at ends of both component bones, capsule, synovial fluid, and synovium. *(B)* In early synovitis, mast cells appear with proliferation of synovium, leading to an increase and change in synovial fluid. *(C)* With an increase of effusion (synovial fluid), there is an increase in polymorphonuclear (PMN) cells and rheumatoid factor IgM. *(D)* The synovium gradually covers the cartilage (forming a pannus). The inflamed synovium secretes lysosomes and lsozymes that erode the cartilage. *(E)* The final stage may be development of fibrous tissue that connects the two denuded cartilaginous surfaces and causes a fibrous fixed joint.

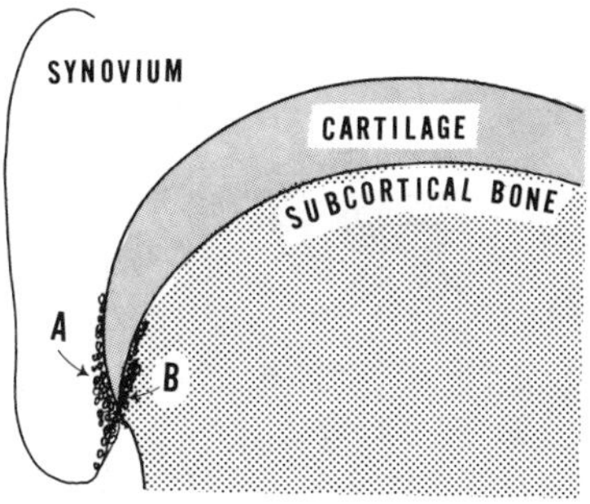

Figure 6-10. Pannus formation of the involved synovium. A depicts the pannus invading the outer area of the cartilage and B the invasion into the area between the cartilage and the subchondral bone.

On examination, the joints are swollen, tender upon palpation, and warm (not hot). The joint feels "boggy" upon palpation. Hand grip strength is diminished. Range of motion is initially limited due to pain and swelling. The superficial tendon may also be swollen and tender.

The course of the disease is highly variable with 15 percent of cases having a complete remission and 10 percent progressing regardless of the proferred treatment. Most patients fall between these two extremes, with periods of remission and periods of exacerbations. Some residual joint impairment and structural damage occurs between "attacks."

Laboratory Findings

Patients demonstrate a normocytic, normochromic anemia and an elevated sedimentation rate (ESR). Approximately 80 percent of patients have a positive rheumatoid factor test. Radiologically, in the early disease, there is noted some osteopenia and soft-tissue swelling. Only in the more advanced stages are the joint spaces affected. Synovial fluid usually shows an elevated white cell count (mostly neutrophils) which varies from 5,000 to 25,000 per cubic millimeter.

Tenosynovitis

Along with the joints, rheumatoid disease affects the tendons. In about two-thirds of all rheumatoid hands there is involvement of the extrinsic tendons.[20] The proliferating synovium of the sheath fills it entirely, adheres to the enclosed tendon and ultimately invades the tendon itself (Fig. 6-11).

The extensor tendons under the extensor retinaculum become involved. As the flexor tendons are enclosed within sheaths they can be involved at many sites along the index, middle, and ring fingers. The

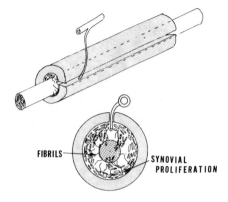

Figure 6–11. Tendonitis. Upper figure depicts a schematic tendon sheath with its two layers. In synovitis, there is an invasion of the inflamed synovium and microfibrils of connective tissue that compresses the tendon and adheres to it.

thumb and little fingers are more susceptible in the portion from the proximal phalanx to the wrist. The five finger flexors tendons are susceptible at the volar tunnel area.

These sites of involvement are used to differentiate rheumatoid arthritis from osteoarthritic changes (Table 6–1).

Due to vascular impairment and synovial invasion, involved tendons may rupture at points of bony pressure or angulation when stretched and cause further articular functional loss. Normally the flexor tendons exert greater mechanical tension and thus are most resilient than extensor tendons, and are less prone to rupture.[21]

Muscles of the Rheumatoid Hand

The extrinsic muscles undergo vasculitis and inflammation. The intrinsic muscles are more vulnerable to concurrent joint and tendon synovitis. The latter undergo protective spasm and by their action cause additional deformity, limitation, and pain.

Table 6–1. COMPARISON OF RHEUMATOID
AND OSTEOARTHROTIC HANDS

	Rheumatoid	*Osteoarthrotic*
Joint involvement	Middle row and metacarpophalangeal	Distal row
Wrist involvement	Usual	Rare if ever
Tenderness	Usual	Rare or minimal
Swelling	Soft of capsule and periarticular	Bony osteophytes

Treatment

The goal of treatment is to reduce the swelling and pain in an attempt to preserve joint function and maintain activities of daily living. Pain can be controlled with anti-inflammatory medications. Narcotics are usually avoided when possible. Salicylates, nonsteroidal anti-inflammatory drugs, low doses of glucocorticoids, gold salts, penicillamine, and methrotrexate, are some of the current mainstays of medical treatment; however, they are not the major focus of this text.

The role of synovectomy, either chemical or surgical in the management of rheumatoid joints of the hand remains controversial.[22]

There are numerous types of inflammatory arthritis such as psoriatic, Reiter's, but only the hand manifestations will be highlighted.

Wrist

No tendons attach to the carpal bones (except the pisiform), but in flexion, extension, radial, and ulnar movement of the hand by the extrinsic muscles, the carpal rows move on each other (see Chapter 1). The carpal bones are united by ligaments; thus when these ligaments are weakened by rheumatoid disease their stability is impaired, and deformity results (Fig. 6–12).

Inflammation and effusion of the carpal joints deform the capsuloligamentous tissues that normally support these joints. The volar ligaments, being stronger than the dorsal, cause imbalance, with resultant stress upon the dorsal aspects of the joints. Attenuation of the ligament binding the distal radial-ulnar articulation causes instability with resultant volar migration of the proximal carpal row and dorsal migration of the distal row (Fig. 6–13).

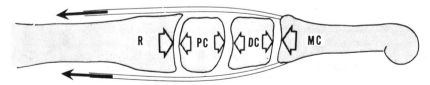

Figure 6–12. Carpal bone stability. With symmetrical dorsal and volar musculotendinous tension, the carpal bones are symmetrically compressed and maintain alignment and stability. Rheumatoid disease can cause imbalance of soft tissue with resultant carpal bone displacement (see Fig. 6–13).

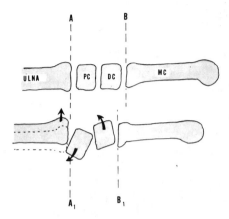

Figure 6–13. Subluxation of carpal bones. Owing to asymmetry of the dorsal and volar musculotendinous pull, the imbalance allows carpal bones to subluxate.

When the extensor carpi ulnaris, which normally passes over the dorsum of the styloid, is frayed, it can slip in a volar direction, become a flexor, and thus pull the fifth metacarpal in a volar direction (Fig. 6–14).

The powerful radial deviators of the hand (extensor carpi radialis longus, extensor carpi radialis brevis, and flexor carpi radialis) are normally overwhelming compared to the ulnar deviators and so cause the hand to deviate radially with the proximal carpal row migrating in an ulnar direction.

The normal ulnar deviation of the hand which is due to the distal alignment of the radius and ulna (Fig. 6–15) causes a compensatory radial deviation of the fingers. When there is overwhelming pull of the proximal carpal row in an ulnar direction, the first metacarpal angle

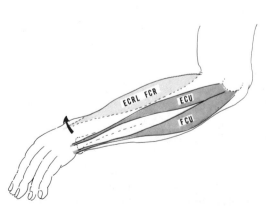

Figure 6–14. Ulnar subluxation of the extensor carpi ulnaris. If the tendon of the extensor carpi ulnaris (ECU) becomes frayed, it can migrate volarly and become a flexor that ulnar-deviates the hand and pulls the fifth metacarpal volarly. A weakened ECU may allow overpull of the radial deviators; the extensor carpi radials longus (ECRL), the extensor carpi radialis brevis, and flexor carpi radialis (FCR).

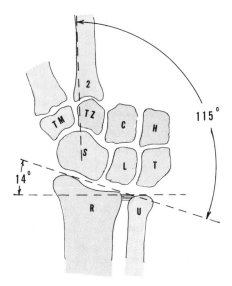

Figure 6–15. Normal alignment of carpal, radial, and metacarpal bones. The distal surface of the radius and ulna usually has an ulnar facing of 14°. The second metacarpal "fixed" to the trapezoid (TZ) is in direct alignment to the radius at a 115° angulation to the distal radial ulnar facing.

changes in a radial direction, furthering the apparent deformity.[23] With the metacarpals deviating in a radial direction the fingers adjust with ulnar deviation.[24]

In the normal situation, there is a physiologic ulnar inclination that occurs at the metacarpophalangeal joints when flexing the hand. This is especially true in the index (second) and middle (third) fingers.[25] This physiologic ulnar drift is related to the 'normal' joint structure and the gradual deformity is probably brought about in the diseased hand from the stress of external forces upon an otherwise normal joint.[26] Ulnar drift does not occur if the intrinsic muscles remain intact, indicating that muscles "can" offer joint stability. The joint ligaments offer the *most* support, and the radial ligaments resisting ulnar deviation are even stronger in the flexed finger position. "Diseased intrinsic muscles are therefore unable to compensate for ligamentous instability."

Passive rotation about the longitudinal axis of the fingers is limited to 15° by the capsule, and the 25° by the collateral ligaments if the capsule is cut. Lateral and medial deviation of the MCP joint is controlled by the ligaments. In power gripping an adduction stress is imposed upon the fingers. The stronger radial collateral ligaments balance these forces over the ulnar ligaments.

It is apparent that in the rheumatoid hand and fingers, careful evaluation of every component of carpal, metacarpal, and phalangeal alignment is needed to correct developing imbalances by appropriate splinting and therapy. Individual hands at varying stages of the disease show the effect of specific and differing deforming forces.[27]

Thumb

The metacarpophalangeal and interphalangeal joints of the thumb move in a flexion-extension direction. Due to the great multidirectional flexibility of the carpometacarpal joint of the thumb, all periarticular ligamentous structures are strong except those on the radial aspect, where the relative weakness allows excessive "adduction." In rheumatoid arthritis, attenuation of the radial ligaments, plus the pull from spasm and contracture of the adductor pollicis, causes the first metacarpal to adduct and flex. Tenodesis action causes the metacarpophalangeal joint to hyperextend and the interphalangeal joint to flex.

There is, however, a propensity of the thumb to develop a boutonniere deformity (Fig. 6–16), in which the MCP joint is flexed and the IP joint hyperextended. This deformity is particularly disabling as it eliminates tip-to-tip pinch and grasp.

Routine examination of the rheumatoid thumb is mandatory as soon as there are signs of acute inflammation. The examination should include circumduction and stability of the carpometacarpal (CMC) joint and the collateral ligaments of the MP and IP joints in the flexed position, when these ligaments are at their tautest. No lateral motion should be elicited.

The thumb at rest should be observed, as well as tip-to-tip action and strength. Each extensor tendon should be evaluated as to its alignment and strength. Early recognition of the condition is mandatory if ultimate deformity and significant impairment to be prevented.

Metacarpophalangeal Joints

The shape of the metacarpophalangeal joint surfaces allows the motions of flexion, extension, some rotation, abduction, and adduction. There is a normal inclination of the proximal phalanx at the MCP joint.

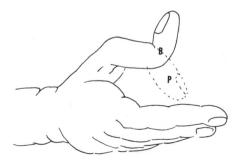

Figure 6–16. Boutonniere deformity of the thumb. The boutonniere deformity with flexion deformity of the metacarpophalangeal joint and interphalangeal hyperextension (B) prevents tip-to-tip (P) opproximation to the index finger.

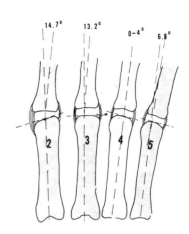

Figure 6–17. Normal inclination angles of proximal phalanx of metacarpophalangeal joints. The recorded angles are the range of abduction-adduction movements of the metacarpophalangeal joints. The differences in lengths of the collateral ligaments are also noted, as are their strengths. The metacarpal heads also have radial facing in the second (2) and third (3) metacarpals and an ulnar facing in the fifth (5) metacarpal. There is *no* angulation of the fourth (4) metacarpal.

This causes a difference in the length of the collateral ligaments (Fig. 6–17) and a variation in the angulation of the distal ends of the metacarpals (Fig. 6–18). Only the fourth (ring) finger is in direct alignment. By virtue of their configuration there is no stability of the metacarpophalangeal joints. Support is afforded essentially by the collateral ligaments and slightly by the capsules.

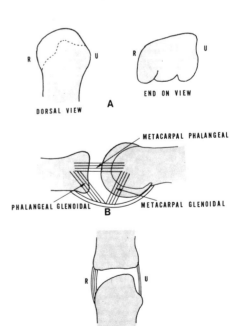

Figure 6–18. Metacarpal distal joint. *(A)* Normal configuration of the metacarpal head. *(B)* Normal ligamentous support of the metacarpophalangeal joint. *(C)* The radial ligament is thicker and attaches more distally; hence, it is longer than the ulnar ligament.

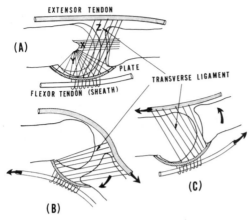

Figure 6–19. Metacarpophalangeal ligaments. *(A)* The collateral ligaments comprise (x) the metacarpophalangeal ligament and (y) the metacarpoglenoidal component, which suspends the palmar plate and in turn the flexor tendons. The check ligament —transverse lamina *(A) (B) (C)*—connects the extensor tendons to the palmar plate and the flexor tendons (see Fig. 1–79) in neutral extension. The metacarpophalangeal ligaments prevent extension bowing; *(B)* in flexion, they are relatively relaxed; and *(C)* they extend the proximal phalanx.

The collateral ligaments of the metacarpophalangeal joints are normally lax in extension, allowing lateral (Fig. 6–19) motion. Because of their unequal length greater ulnar deviation is permitted. The difference in the insertions of the radial and ulnar intrinsic muscles (Fig. 6–20) into the extensor mechanisms also favors ulnar deviation in the normal hand, as does the fact that there is an ulnar bend of the flexor tendon at the MP joint (Fig. 6–21).

The force required (Fig. 6–22) on the flexor tendon during tip pinch is estimated as being six times the pinching force at the finger tip. With 30° of flexion at the MP joint the force placed upon the volar aspect of the ligament is three times the pinch force, and the force towards ulnar deviation is twice as great.[28]

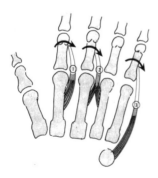

① 1st PALMAR INTEROSSEOUS
② 3rd DORSAL INTEROSSEOUS   ⇨ "SPASM"
③ ABDUCTOR DIGITI QUINTI

Figure 6–20. Ulnar drift caused by selective intrinsic muscle spasm, then contracture.

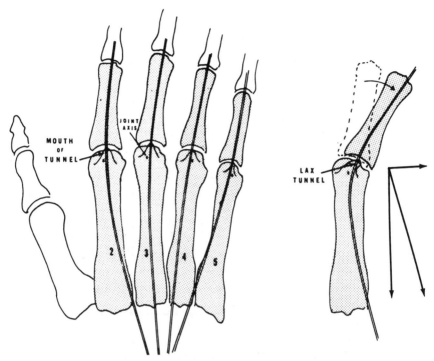

Figure 6–21. Mechanism of ulnar deviation (flexor concept). Normally, the flexor tendons enter the tunnel of the flexor pulley, which has a taut mouth. The tendons then veer in an ulnar direction. In the index (2) and middle (3) fingers, the tendon passes to the ulnar side of the joint axis. The tendons (4) and (5) pass radial to axis. Normally, the phalanges deviate ulnarly. In rheumatoid disease, the mouth of the tunnel becomes lax, permitting the flexor tendons to veer more ulnarly.

Figure 6–22. Mechanism of volar subluxation of metacarpophalangeal joint. (1) The normal pulley assembly fulcrums the flexor tendons during a forceful pinch. The normal mouth of the tunnel is the flexor pulley. (2) In rheumatoid arthritis, the tunnel and its mouth are frayed and elongated, permitting the flexor tendon to move volarly, thus causing the volar force to sublux the phalanx upon the metacarpal head. The metacarpophalangeal collateral ligaments are also relaxed, permitting this subluxation as well as ulnar deviation.

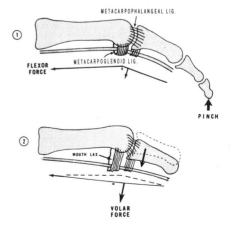

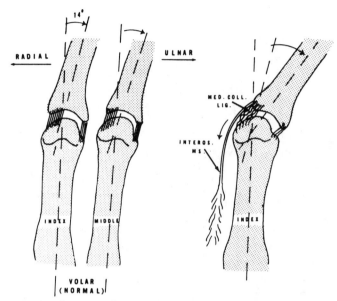

Figure 6–23. Mechanism of ulnar deviation of digits in rheumatoid arthritis. The normal hand finds ulnar deviation of the metacarpophalangeal of an average of 14°. This is most prevalent in the index and second middle fingers. In rheumatoid arthritis, the collateral ligaments, especially the radial side, weaken and lengthen. The intrinsic muscles are unable to compensate for this deviation and ulnar shift results.

It becomes apparent that forces and structures all lead to ulnar deviation, and when there is weakening of these structures from inflammation the disparity becomes greater. Weakening of the collateral ligaments (Fig. 6–23), the flexion forces of the intrinsic muscles, as well as the extrinsic forces, cause volar subluxation and ultimate dislocation of the joints.

All involved structures and forces must be constantly evaluated in the rheumatoid hand to intervene at an appropriate time.

Proximal Interphalangeal Joints

These joints normally flex and extend but do not physiologically hyperextend, nor do they deviate laterally. The palmar plates of this joint are restrictive and the metacarpophalangeal and the metacarpoglenoid ligaments are reinforced by the retinacular ligaments that connect the extensor mechanism to the flexor mechanisms (see Fig. 6–19).

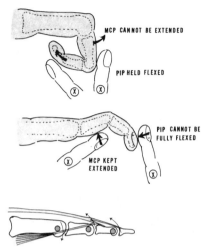

MCP CANNOT BE EXTENDED

PIP HELD FLEXED

PIP CANNOT BE FULLY FLEXED

MCP KEPT EXTENDED

Figure 6–24. Spasm of intrinsics. The metacarpophalangeal joint becomes flexed as does the proximal interphalangeal joint. If the metacarpophalangeal joint is passively extended, the interphalangeal joints cannot be flexed fully. Bottom illustration depicts the normal attachments and action upon the finger joints.

The proximal interphalangeal joint is frequently involved in rheumatoid arthritis and may decide whether a boutonniere deformity or swan neck deformity occurs.

In summary the joint changes causing characteristic deformities are:

Ulnar Deviation: Laxity of the MP joint capsules and collateral ligaments with movement of the extensor and flexor tendons in an ulnar direction. The intrinsic muscles become tight (Fig. 6–24).

Ulnar deviation may be cosmetically unpleasant but not necessarily functionally disabling. Most grip functions are retained if flexion is retained. The greatest functional loss is extension of the fingers resulting from dislocation of the extensor mechanism. In "severe" ulnar deviation the tip-to-tip grip of the thumb and index finger may be lost as it is in boutonniere deformity.

The mechanism of ulnar deviation of the little finger remains conjectural. One theory is that the abductor digit minimi becomes overwhelming or unopposed. Also the hypothenar muscles attach to the ulnar side and are considered stronger than the palmar interrossei and lumbicals on the radial side. This ulnar deviation also impairs finger tip-to-tip activities.

Boutonniere Deformity: Laxity of the PIP joint capsule, volar movement of the lateral bands, shortening of the oblique retinacular ligaments, and some elongation of the central extensor tendon (Fig. 6–25).

This deformity is difficult to treat as no functional splint has been found to be effective, and surgical intervention has also been unsatisfactory (Fig. 6–26).

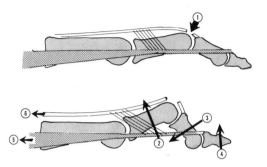

Figure 6-25. Boutonniere deformity. There is a stretch or tear (1) of the central extensor slip. The lateral bands migrate volarly (2) and flex the proximal interphalangeal joints (3). The distal phalanx extends (4) and the intrinsics (5) and extensors (6) migrate proximally.

Swan Neck Deformity: Flexor tenosynovitis with laxity of the PIP joint capsule and the accessory collateral ligaments, dorsal movement of the lateral bands, lengthening of the oblique retinacular ligaments and synovitis of the flexor tendon (Fig. 6-27).

This deformity occurs in approximately 28 percent of rheumatoid arthritis cases.[29] The metacarpophalangeal joint subluxes in a volar direction owing to the spasm and ultimate contracture of the intrinsic muscles. The proximal interphalangeal joint extends.

This deformity can be averted with proper splinting (Fig. 6-28) to limit or prevent hyperextension of the interphalangeal joint before contracture occurs. Worn day and night it permits the palmar plates and collateral ligaments to take up the slack and maintains the integrity of the flexor mechanism.

Mallet Deformity: Laxity of the DIP (distal inter-phalangeal) capsule and rupture or stretch of the extensor tendon (Fig. 6-29). Splinting is effective if the treatment is applied "before" there is contracture or subluxation. Surgical intervention is often indicated to prevent con-

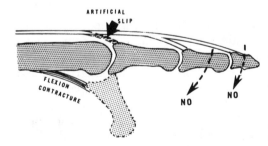

Figure 6-26. Surgical treatment of the metacarpophalangeal flexion deformity. The construction of an artificial slip to the proximal phalanx to assist extension also impairs flexion of the two distal digits. The flexion contracture is one of the disabling aspects of rheumatoid arthritis. If the extensor is anchored with fingers flexed (the proximal and distal interphalangeal joints), all long extensor action must be done by the intrinsics, which must be normal in insertion as well as innervation. This normalcy can hardly be expected in rheumatoid arthritis.

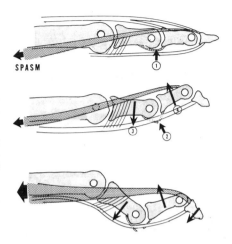

Figure 6–27. Swan neck deformity. Spasm, then contracture of the intrinsic muscles causes hyperextension (4) of the middle phalanx. The volar pouch synovitis causes laxity (1) of the proximal interphalangeal joint with ultimate disruption (2). As the intrinsics move dorsal to the axis of rotation, the proximal phalanx flexes (3). Traction, resulting from tenodesis action upon the distal phalanx, causes the distal phalanx to flex.

tinued deformity and impairment (Fig. 6–30) of the mallet finger at this stage, before there is contracture or subluxation.

Inflammatory Tendon Diseases

In rheumatoid diseases the involvement of tendons can present significant pathology, pain, functional impairment. Of these tendon conditions the following are the most prevalent:

1. "Snapping" tendons.
2. Stenosis of tendons within their sheaths.
3. Rupture of tendons.

Some of these conditions have already been mentioned. In rheumatoid disease, there is a tendency for nodules to form within the tendons.

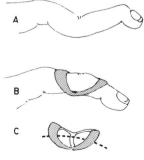

Figure 6–28. Splint for swan neck deformity. Before contracture or subluxation occurs, the swan neck deformity (A) can be held or minimized by the simple splint shown in C. This splint limits hyperextension of the proximal interphalangeal joint and permits flexion of this joint (B). (Adapted from Licht S, ed.: Arthritis and Physical Medicine. Elizabeth Licht, Publisher, New Haven, 1969, with permission.)

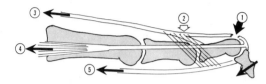

Figure 6–29. Mallet finger. A rupture or tear of the extensor tendon (1) primal to the insertion of the lateral bands (2) upon the proximal aspect of the distal phalanx allows horizontal proximal pull of the extendor tendon (3) upon the flexor digitorum profundus tendon (5), thus flexing the distal phalanx.

These nodules are a retraction of the torn afflicted collagen fibers that "bunch" into a nodule (Fig. 6–31). These torn fibers weaken the tendon and predispose it to tearing as well as bunching. The nodularity prevents free movement within the usual tight sheath and results in "snapping" when movement of the tendon is momentarily restricted at an angulation. These snapping tendons, also called "trigger fingers," can be both heard and felt, and are restrictive of daily finger function.

Examination of a tendon that is constricted due to nodularity indicates the presence of a palpabale nodule or of a "snapping" that can be felt or heard during flexion of that joint.

Treatment of a snapping tendon involves injection into the sheath of a soluble steroid to increase the lubrication and/or decrease the inflammation of the tendon, in hope of decreasing the size of the nodule or increasing the capacity of the sheath. If the nodule is extensive or intractable, the sheath may be incised or the nodule excised. Either may result in a weakened tendon that ultimately may tear and result in loss or impairment of joint function.

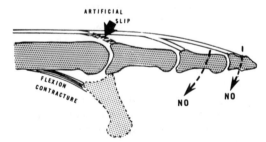

Figure 6–30. Surgical treatment of the metacarpophalangeal flexion deformity. The construction of an artificial slip to the proximal phalanx to assist extension also impairs flexion of the two distal digits. The flexion contracture is one of the disabling aspects of rheumatoid arthritis. If the extensor is anchored with fingers flexed (the proximal and distal interphalangeal joints), all long extensor action must be done by the intrinsics, which must be normal in insertion as well as innervation. This normalcy can hardly be expected in rheumatoid arthritis.

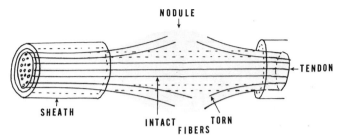

Figure 6-31. Formation of a tendon nodule. The parallel collagen fibers of a tendon become "torn" from disease, attritition, or trauma. The tendency of a collagen is to retract thus the torn fibers retract to form a nodule. The tendon which is tightly contained within its sheath thus becomes larger than the sheath and either is restricted in motion or "snaps" when the nodule attempts to pass by the constricted area of sheath.

Evaluation Of Functional Impairment

While the evaluation and the ensuing treatment of rheumatoid articular or tendon disease is directed to function, the evaluation of malfunction must obviously be a major component of history and examination.

In evaluating the rheumatoid hand all "grips" must be examined, and limited or defective grips must be analyzed as to the joint capsule, articular damage, muscle and/or tendon involved. Impairment of an individual joint of a single finger does not constitute functional loss.

There are four basic hand positions and functions that must be evaluated:

1. Grip 1 is a tip-to-tip pinch of the index finger to the thumb (Fig. 6-32, top). This pinch grip requires abduction of the thumb flexion of the index finger at the proximal interphalangeal joint. This is a precision grip used to manipulate small objects or to initiate precision activities.
2. Grip 2 is a more powerful grip (Fig. 6-32), in which the thumb presses against the side of the index finger. All the joints of the thumb and fingers must be free and the intrinsic muscles (first dorsal interossei, adductor pollicis, and so on) strong.
3. Grip 3 is used for grasping objects having a handle, such as a knife, screwdriver, or scissors. (Fig. 6-33, top). In this grip not only must grip 2 be free and strong but the object must be steadied pressure of the ring and little finger toward the thenar eminence. Loss of flexion of the little (fifth) finger is a severe impairment of the grip.

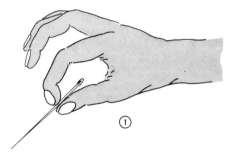

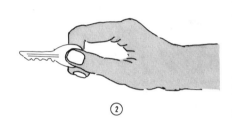

Figure 6–32. Various grips of op-position. (1) Tip-to-tip opposition is functional and precise, requiring opposition of the thumb and rotation of the index finger in an ulnar direction (see Fig. 1–69). (2) The key grip requires adduction of the thumb and no rotation of the fingers.

4. Grip 4 is a "pistol grip" Fig. 6–33, bottom). In addition to the power aspects of grips 2 and 3, all fingers must adequately flex to form a "hook," and the thumb must adduct to form an area against which to press.

In the early phase of rheumatoid arthritis there is an acute inflammation of the joints, tendons, and intrinsic muscles, yet all remain functional within limits. The swelling of any joint limits range of motion, and inflammation and/or spasm of the intrinsic muscles limits active motion. If there is persistent inflammation, or when the acute inflammation has subsided, the resultant deformity must be evaluated. These deformities include joint subluxation, contracture of muscle and/or joint, and tendon disruption.

Loss of joint flexion is, as a rule, more disabling than is the loss of extension. All four grips require adequate flexion. Thus in loss or impairment of a specific grip action, all involved joints, tendons, and muscles must be evaluated.

The carpometacarpal joint of the ring and little finger normally has a limited flexion range, but loss of this range of motion presents a severe disability, especially in grips 3 and 4. Ankylosis of these joints in a flexed position is not disabling.

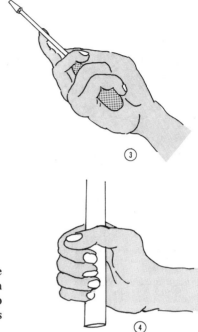

Figure 6-33. Wrist-finger grips. The precision grip (3) requires ulnar deviation of the hand and fingers. The power grip (4) is used for such activities as hammering.

The metacarpophalangeal joints normally flex 90°. Loss of a few degrees of flexion in the ring and little fingers causes significant functional impairment. Loss of flexion in the index and middle fingers is usually less significant functionally. Even severe subluxation or ulnar deviation, or both, usually does not result in functional impairment.

The proximal interphalangeals joints normally flex to more than 90° and minor loss is usually well tolerated. In the ring and little fingers the critical point in flexion is 120°. Loss of flexion to 120° results in functional loss. Significant loss of flexion of all fingers results in loss of grip 4. In swan neck deformities due to hyperextension complex (see Fig. 6-27) there is a loss of flexion that results in disability.

Functional loss from loss of extension is uncommon, unless the loss is extreme. Most normal extension occurs at the metacarpophalangeal and proximal interphalangeal joints, thus loss of extension merely prevents the hand from holding or grasping large objects. If firm, fixed flexion contractures cause the loss or impaired extension, the functional loss may be significant. Severe flexion deformities are rare in the proximal interphalangeal joints.

Ulnar deviation, while cosmetically undesirable, is not a severe disability unless there is also a loss of metacarpophalangeal flexion. In severe ulnar deviation there is a weakness of grip between the thumb and index finger (grip 1, Fig. 6–32, top).

Palmar subluxation or dislocation often occurs simultaneously with ulnar deviation and is considered as an ulnar deviation, since both are aggravated by forceful flexion. Subluxation of the extensor tendons occurs as a result (not a cause) of ulnar deviation. Although it is not considered a "cause," once established, extensor activity increases the ulnar deviation. This subluxation initially occurs in the little finger and "spreads" to the middle finger.

General Concepts of Treatment

The ultimate goal in the management of rheumatoid arthritis is to maintain or improve function in the activities of daily living and/or occupation. These activities demand a functional assessment both subjective and active.[30]

The general goals of conservative management are to alleviate inflammation and pain, maintain stability and mobility of joints by preserving the articular and periarticular tissues, and maintaining muscle-tendon function. Management of inflammation and resultant pain is approached by the application of specific modalities.[31,32]

Neither heat nor cold affect the basic pathology or provide long-term benefits,[33] but they assist in the performance of therapeutic exercises and enhance the comfort to the patient.

Splints do not prevent deformity when the disease is progressing, but they do minimize pain, protect the inflamed joints from excessive internal and external traumatic forces, and permit continuation of daily activities.

Splints can be considered as "static" or "kinetic," each with a precise indication and function. A precaution that must be considered is their effect on contiguous joints, this effect may be beneficial or adverse. Splints should not enhance muscular atrophy, nor enhance joint contracture. A careful examination the involved joint(s) and their functional loss will determine the precise functional need for the splint and determine the material and structure of the orthotics.

Dynamic splints should provide gentle prolonged force to stretch the involved soft tissue and afford resistance to the weakened muscles being exercised. Dynamic splints may control or guide motion, and obviate adverse action.

Exercises are indicated to maintain or regain range of motion and/or muscle strength and endurance. The purpose of any exercise is the basis for the prescription. Whether the prescribed exercise should be active or passive is decided after careful assessment of the impairment and the precise tissue.

Rest between exercises is paramount in the presence of active inflammation and must be carefully noted in the prescription. The duration, frequency, and intensity of any exercise must also be accurately designated.[34] "Respect pain" is a meaningful principle.[35]

OSTEOARTHRITIS

Degenerative arthritis, osteoarthritis, or osteoarthrosis is a common disorder affecting many joints of the human body, including the hand. It is a condition known in antiquity, yet still eluding full understanding as to etiology. It may not have the ominous portent of rheumatoid arthritis, yet it causes pain, impairs function, and presents cosmetic deformity. The common label of "benign arthropathy of inevitable aging" has been of little comfort to the affected patient.

Mechanisms

Before progressing to a discussion of the possible cause of the "degeneration" of human cartilage, the structure, chemistry, and function of normal cartilage can be beneficially reviewed. The nutrition of cartilage is maintained by the infusion and diffusion of fluids (Fig. 6–34). The structure of normal cartilage makes this nutrition possible in that normal cartilage is composed of collagen fibers within a matrix. The collagen fibers are coiled, allowing them to act as compression "springs." Compression causes flattening of the cartilage and relaxation permits expansion; together they cause mechanical "inhibition."

Articular cartilage consists of cellular and extracellular components. The extracellular components are collagen, proteoglycans, and other proteins; the cellular components are chondrocytes (5% of the volume). Collagen types are an active area of research. Currently 14 types of collagen have been found in the body, with types II, IX, X, and XI being found in cartilage.

The proteoglycan matrix is negatively charged and is hydrophilic, having a strong affinity for water. The matrix encourages diffusion of nutrients, and the enclosed collagen fibers afford tensile strength.

Collagen fibers have been described earlier, in Chapter 4 (Figs. 4–1 to Fig. 4–3.) The collagen molecule is composed of three polypeptide chains (α chains) (Fig. 4–1), in which every third residue is the amino acid glycine and the others, X and Y, are often proline and hydroxyproline respectively. Each chain (trihelix) is connected to its

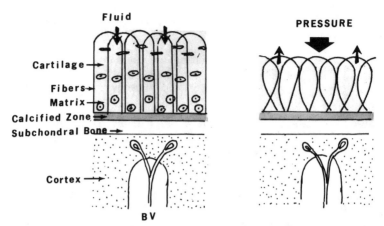

Figure 6–34. Cartilage nutrition. (Left) The "relaxed" cartilage has collagen fibers and chondrocyte cells within the matrix. These cells are active in the basal layers and flatten toward the periphery until they become flat and flake off when they exit the cartilage. The zone immediately below the cartilage is the calcified zone that does not permit the passage of blood vessels (BV) into the cartilage. Immediately under this zone is the subchondral bone and then the cortex. The blood vessels end as bulbs. In the relaxed state the cartilage is expanded and absorbs fluid (small arrows) from the synovial cavity. (Right) The cartilage is compressed by gravity and muscular contraction (large arrow). This occurs because of compression of the collagen fiber "springs." Fluid is compressed from the cartilage to "weep" into the synovial cavity (small arrows).

adjacent chain by an interchain hydrogen bond (proline hydroxy group.)[36] These intermolecular cross-links are also the sites of gylcosylation which are involved in nutrition and remodeling.

The structure of type IX collagen fibers differs fundamentally from that of type II fibers and is considered to be the "glue" which holds all the type II fibers together (Fig. 6–35). Its degradation is also consid-

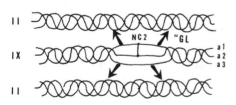

Figure 6–35. The role of Type IX collagen in cartilage. There are predominantly Type II, IX, X, and XI collagen fibers in cartilage. Genetically determined Type IX has been hypothesized as being the "glue" that holds the Type II fibers together. Degradation leading to degenerative changes has been thought to represent "ungluing" of the collagen weakening the structure of the cartilage. What causes ungluing remains obscure.

ered to be the basis for degenerative arthritic conditions. As the type of collagen fiber is genetically determined this may be a clue as to why degenerative arthritis is present in some people and not others, that is, there may be predisposition to DJD. Genetic factors are dominant in women and recessive in men, which may account for the predominance of DJD in women.

Degradation of articular cartilage occurs as a result of the release of proteolytic enzymes from chondrocytes, synovial cells, and neutrophils.[37] These proteinases are termed collagenase (destroys collagen), stromelysin (destroys matrix), and neutrophil elastase (destroys elastin). These enzymes are allegedly regulated by an inhibitor metalloproteinase (TIMP). When there is an imbalance between TIMP and the proteinases, degenerative changes occur in the cartilage.[38] What causes this imbalance remains conjectural, but the result is that type IX fibers are disrupted and the "glue" between type II fibers is weakened.

Normal cartilage tends to deform in such a way as to cause tension at its marginal periphery. A constant clinical finding is the presence of cartilage degeneration in the load-bearing areas. This implies that compression and shear play a vital role in degeneration. Cartilage is too thin to be an effective shock absorber in spite of its viscoelastic properties.

Cartilage absorbs most of the shock at its bony union, which deforms upon compression, and through the external forces of the musculoligamentous reaction (see Fig. 4–3). How this external neuromuscular stress reaction of cartilage affects the cartilaginous degeneration is not clear, but it must be considered a pertinent factor.

Whether or not the surface of cartilage continues to be slowly worn away during life is also conjectural (Fig. 6–36). Repeated oscillation and longitudinal loading probably leads (Fig. 6–37) to "fatigue" of cartilage, with resultant mechanical and chemical changes. The effect of friction upon cartilage has been declared as "negligible."[39,40]

The lubricant expressed from cartilage under pressure is hyaluronic acid. It minimizes friction but also acts as an "adhesive" keeping the articular surface together.

Compression of cartilage flattens the coiled collagen fibers, whereas shear, which is a recurrent force impressed upon active joints, deforms the angulation of the fibers (see Fig. 6–34).

To summarize, the degenerative changes result from:

1. Longitudinal forces including mechanical impact and muscular contraction.
2. Compressive forces upon the cartilage.
3. Impact upon the subchondral bone with resultant microfractures.

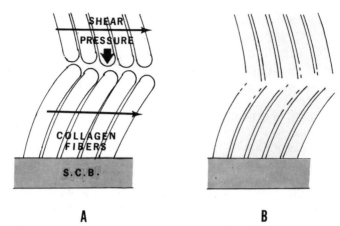

A   **B**

Figure 6–36. Shear deformation of cartilage. *(A)* The opposing cartilages of a moving joint cause the curving deformation of the collagen fibers. This shear force is augmented by compressive forces from gravity and muscular action. The underlying subchondral one (S.C.B.) is shown. *(B)* The shear effect has caused a degeneration of the collagen fiber with irregularity of the cartilage matrix.

These traumata alter the metabolism of the cartilage.[41] They change the pore size of the matrix components and cause an outflow of matrix, so as to alter the osmotic pressure of the cartilage. The matrix is also altered by the action of lysosomal lytic enzymes.

Studies on trauma to cartilage have focused on the repair mechanisms that follow lacerations (Fig. 6–38) in laboratory animals. Superficial lacerations not approaching the subchondral bone do not progress nor do they heal. Deep lacerations that violate the underlying bone plate undergo characteristic changes (Fig. 6–38).

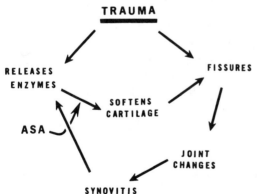

Figure 6–37. Schematic of the processes that help cause degenerative arthritis.

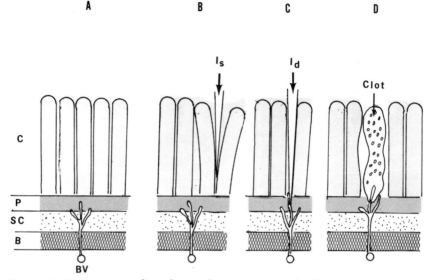

Figure 6 – 38. Response of cartilage to laceration to study the response to injury. *(A)* Normal cartilage (C) with a calcified plate (P), subchondral bone (SC), and bone cortex *(B)* that contains the blood vessels (BV). *(B)* A shallow laceration (I_S) that does not reach the subchondral bone. Healing does not occur, nor is there progression of the damage. *(C)* A deep laceration (I_D) that penetrates matrix and enters the subchondral bone plate. The blood vessels (BV) enter the area of laceration. *(D)* Repair with the penetrated blood vessels forming a blood clot that contains cells and fibroblasts. This heals into a fibrocartilaginous tissue.

Initially the defect fills with blood cells from the end plate blood vessels and the cells immediately become organized into a fibrous clot. Within 10 days some of the blood cells change into fibroblasts. With chondrification, "fibrocartilage" tissue is formed and fills the defect forming a "dimple" within the surrounding normal cartilage.

Chemical changes occur, including an increase in the concentration of proteolytic enzymes within the degenerating cartilage,[42] where the concentration of proteoglycans diminishes and their chemical characteristics alter.[43] For unknown reasons there occurs an increase in water content.

Initially, in degenerative cartilage changes, flaking of the superficial surface is noted. This occurs to a greater degree in cartilage that has been predisposed by trauma, genetic, hormonal and/or metabolic enzymic influences. Cysts form in the tangential layers that open into the joint surfaces and form larger craters (Fig. 6 – 39). Hyaluronidase and other enzymes penetrate into these craters, causing loss of chondroitin, which is a component of cartilage matrix. Loss of elasticity results, and

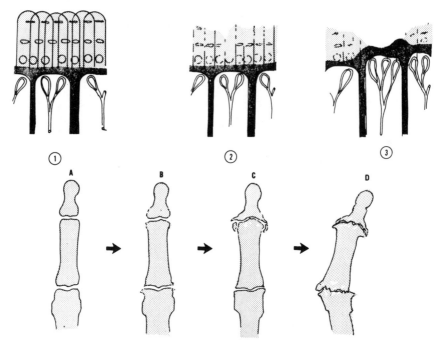

Figure 6–39. Natural history of degenerative osteoarthrosis. (1) Normal cartilage through stress undergoes alteration of cartilage surface. (2) Penetration of synovial hyaluronidase into cartilage causes degeneration of the matrix. Collagen fibers erode as does the cartilage. Subhcondral vascularity increases, causing proliferation of bone into the denuded cartilage areas (3). A through D, Typical x-ray results show changes from normal finger joints to early lipping of joint margins, with gradual formation of periarticular ossicles and severe erosion with subarticular cysts and the obliteration of the joint spaces.

the synovial lubricants lose their viscosity, add both of which further mechanical trauma to the joint. As there is progressive loss of cartilage the subchondral bone fills the denuded areas until the opposing joint surfaces are separated by bone, fibrocartilage, and decreasing normal cartilage.

There are three types of degenerative arthritis involved in the hand:

1. Primary arthritis, in which there is distal interphalangeal joint involvement only. In these cases there may be swelling, pain, and impairment. Heberden's nodes evolve. Usually considered a sequel of aging, this type of arthritis can occur in young people if there is a familial predisposition

2. Generalized osteoarthritis, in which there is involvement of many joints in the body. In the hand, the distal interphalangeal joints are predominantly involved as is thumb carpometacarpal joint.
3. Erosive osteoarthritis, in which the distal and proximal joints undergo progressive destruction.

Treatment

The acutely painful joint can be benefited by the local rest offered by splinting. Usually, two weeks of splinting affords relief. Intra-articular injection of an analgesic anesthetic agent with steroids also gives good respite from pain and inflammation (Fig. 6–40). This relief may be brief, but in many cases has significant duration to justify repeated injection. Salicylates are often beneficial, but the newer nonsteroidal drugs may be needed for relief. Heat in the form of warm water is beneficial and avoiding any movements that are painful is helpful.

Patients with osteoarthritis must be taught to live with their illness. The joints must be kept limber; therefore, in spite of discomfort, all involved joints must be moved frequently. Heat treatment preceding exercises makes them more tolerable. The exercises are designed to prevent stiffness, and for this, heat is beneficial. Passive exercises (those administered to the patient) are rarely necessary, but active assistive exercises may be considered when a joint is becoming limited and contracted.

Surgery may be indicated for patients with painful disabling joints. Surgical candidates must be carefully selected. They must have full knowledge of the problem, full understanding of the procedure, and acceptance that the surgery will ameliorate but *not* restore normal function or appearance to the hand.

The most frequent procedure recommended is that of fusion of the involved joint, usually the distal interphalangeal joint. Fusion restores a

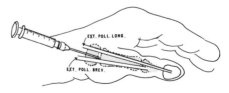

Figure 6–40. Treatment of arthritis of the trapeziometacarpal joint by steroid injection technique. The joint can be felt medial to the elevation of the base of the first metacarpal. Flexing the thumb into the palm opens the joint more. The needle is inserted just lateral to the extensor pollicis brevis within the confines of the snuff formed by the two extensor pollicis tendons.

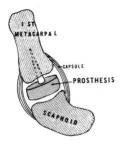

Figure 6–41. Silicone prosthesis for trapezium replacement. This prosthesis requires an adequate capsule and thus must be done early after resection.

functional position, removes undesirable cosmetic deformities, and relieves pain. Fusion may be performed by insertion of a K-wire after resection of the involved articular cartilage. The wire remains for approximately eight weeks, along with an external splint. The proximal joints must be moved.

Surgery may be considered for pain at the base of the thumb if conservative measures have failed to give relief. (Fig. 6–41). Although fusion of the base of the thumb (carpometacarpal joint) may provide a pain-free joint, this technique requires prolonged immobilization which may be unacceptable and can cause disuse atrophy or limitation of contiguous joints. A joint considered for fusion must be splinted preoperatively to allow the patient to experience the loss of movement and to accept that functional limitation.

Excision of the trapezius may relieve pain, but it shortens the thumb and decreases its strength (Fig. 6–42). Joints tend to become unstable after excision arthroplasty. The choice is a matter of the surgeon's experience and the patient's specific need.

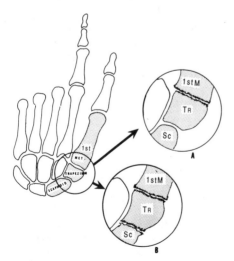

Figure 6–42. Surgical indication for arthritis of the trapeziometacarpal joint (A). Arthritis of the first carpometacarpal joint may require surgical intervention. These procedures consist of excision of the trapezium or fusion of the trapeziometacarpal joint. Excision of the trapezium gives relief of pain but carries danger of resultant weakness of grip. Arthrodesis gives relief of pain unless there is arthritic change in the trapezioscaphoid joint (B).

Some degenerative changes in joints contiguous to the carpophalangeal joint of the thumb may cause pain and disability. The trapezioscaphoid joint may undergo degeneration, along with changes in the carpophalangeal joint of the thumb (see Fig. 6–42). These changes, themselves painful, may persist after successful treatment of the carpophalangeal joint.

When the trapezioscaphoid joint becomes inflamed, the flexor carpi radialis tendon, which passes near it, may also become inflamed. If, with the underlying joint inflammation, synovial fluid escapes into the tendon sheath, a ganglion may be formed. This palmar ganglion occurs infrequently, but, when present, its relationship to underlying degenerative joint disease can be verified by an arthrogram. The results will show that dye injected into the trapezioscaphoid joint seeps into the ganglion.

There are replacement prostheses for the proximal interphalangeal joints. If surgery is ultimately indicated, it should be performed by a qualified hand surgeon.

REFERENCES

1. Thomas CL (ed): Taber's Cyclopedic Medical Dictionary, ed 16. FA Davis, Philadelphia, 1989, p 1733.
2. Tillman LJ, Cummings GS: Biological mechanisms of connective tissue mutability. In Dean P. Currier, Nelson RM. (eds): Dynamics of Human Biological Tissues. FA Davis, Philadelphia, 1992, p 1–44.
3. Cailliet R: Soft Tissue Pain and Disability, ed 2. FA Davis, Philadelphia, 1988.
4. Cailliet R: Pain: Mechanisms and Management, ed 1. FA Davis, Philadelphia, 1993.
5. Connolly JF: DePalma's The Management of Fractures and Dislocations, Vol 2. WB Saunders, Philadelphia, 1981, p 1008.
6. Hunt TK, Banda MJ, Silver IA: Cell interactions in post traumatic fibrosis. Clin Symp 114:128–149, 1985.
7. Tsukamoto Y, Helsel WE, Wahl SM: Macrophage production of fibronectin, a chemattractant for fibroblasts. J Immunol 127:673–678, 1981.
8. Bush DC: Dislocations of the small joints of the hand—simple and complex. In Cowen NJ (ed): Practical Hand Surgery. Yearbook Medical, Chicago, 1980, p 295.
9. Posner MA: Carpal bone dislocations and fractures. In Chapman MW, Madison M (eds): Operative Orthopaedics. JB Lippincott, Philadelphia, 1988, p 1251.
10. Frykman SF, Nelson EF: Fractures and traumatic conditions of the wrist. In Hunter JM et al. (eds): Rehabilitation of the Hand, ed 3. CV Mosby, St. Louis 1990, p 267.
11. Mennel J: The Science and Art of Joint Manipulation, ed 2, Vol 1. J & A Churchill, London, 1949, p 13.
12. Stanley B: Therapeutic exercise: maintaining and restoring mobility in the hand (eds): In Stanley BG, Tribuzi SM (eds): Concepts in Hand Rehabilitation, FA Davis, Philadelphia, 1992, p 178–215.
13. Eaton RG: Joint Injuries of the Hand. Charles C Thomas, Springfield, Ill., 1971.
14. Cannon NM et al,: Diagnosis and Treatment Manual for Physicians and Therapists, ed 2. Hand Rehabilitation Center, Indianapolis, 1985.

15. Watson HK, Maglana W: Complications of fracture management of the hand and wrist. In Gossling HR, Pillsbury SL (eds): Complications of Fracture Management. JB Lippincott, Philadelphia, 1984, p 389.
16. Stark RH: Treatment of difficult PIP fractures with mini-external fixation device. Orthop Rev: 12:609–615, 1993.
17. Gilliland BC: Arthritis and periarthritic disorders. In: Bonica J: The Management of Pain, ed 2, Vol. 1. Lea & Febiger, Philadelphia, 1990, p 329.
18. Cailliet R: Mechanisms of joints. In Licht S (ed): Arthritis and Physical Medicine, Vol 11. Elizebeth Licht, 1969, pp 17–34.
19. MacConaill MA: The movements of bones and joints. J Bone Joint Surg (Br) 32B:244–252, 1950.
20. Flatt AE: The Care of the Rheumatoid Hand, ed 2. CV Mosby, St Louis, 1968.
21. Staub LR, Wilson EH: Spontaneous rupture of extensor tendons in the hand associated with rheumatoid arthritis. J Bone Joint Surg (Am) 38A:1208, 1965.
22. Goldie IF: Synovectomy in rheumatoid arthritis: a general review and an eight year follow-up of synovectomy in fifty rheumatoid patients. Semin Arthritis Rheum, 3: 219–251, 1974.
23. Robinson HS, Kokan PJ, MacBain KP, Patterson FP: Functional results of excisional arthroplasty for the rheumatoid hand. Can Med J, 108:1495–1499, 1978
24. Vaughn-Jackson OJ: Attrition ruptures of tendons as a factor in the production of deformities of the rheumatoid hand. Proc R Soc Med 52:132, 1959
25. Brewerton DA: Hand deformities in rheumatoid disease. Ann Rheum Dis 16:183, 1957.
26. Shapiro JS: A new factor in the etiology of ulnar drift. Clin Orthop 68:32, 1970.
27. Marx H: Rheumatoid arthritis, In Stanley BG, Tribuzi SM (eds): Concepts in Hand Rehabilitation. FA Davis, Philadelphia, 1992 pp 395–418,
28. Smith EM et al.: Flexor forces and rheumatoid metacarpophalangeal deformity. JAMA 198:150–154, 1966.
29. Backhouse KM: The mechanics of normal digital control in the hand and an analysis of the ulnar drift of rhematoid arthritis. Ann R Coll Surg 43:154, 1968.
30. The Professional Staff Association of the Rancho Los Amigos Hospital: Upper Extremity Surgeries for Patients with Rheumatoid Arthritis, A Pre- and Post-operative Treatment Guide. RLAH, Downey, Calif, 1979.
31. Cailliet R: Pain: Mechanisms and Management, FA Davis, Philadelphia, 1993.
32. Michlovitz S: The use of heat and cold in the management of rheumatic diseases. In Michlovitz S (ed): Thermal Agents in Rehabilitation, ed 2. FA Davis, Philadelphia, 1986.
33. Banwell BF: Therapeutic head and cold. In Riggs GK, Gall EP (eds): Rheumatic Diseases, Rehabilitation and Management. Butterworth, Boston, 1984.
34. Wickersham B, Schweidler H: Arthritis—Self Study Guide for Physical and Occupational Therapists. Southwest Arthritis Center, Tucson, 1983.
35. Melvin J: Rheumatic Diseases—Occupational Therapy and Rehabilitation. FA Davis, Philadelphia, 1983.
36. Diab M: The role of type IX collagen in osteoarthritis and rheumatoid arthritis. Orthop Rev 165–170, 1993.
37. Polle AR: Enzymic degradation: cartilage destruction. In Brandt KD (ed): Cartilage Changes in Osteoarthritis, Indiana University School Medicine, Indianapolis, 1990, pp 63–72.
38. Dean DD, Martel-Pelletier J, Pelletier J-P et al.: Evidence for metalloproteinase and metalloproteinase-inhibitor imbalance in human osteoarthritic cartilage. J Clin Invest 84:678–685, 1989.
39. Smith JW: Observations on the postural mechanisms of the human knee joint. J Anat 90:236, 1956.

40. Johns RJ, Wright V: Relative importance of various tissues in joint stiffness, J Appl Physiol 17:824, 1962.
41. Coutts RD: Symposium: the diagnosis and treatment of injuries involving the articular cartilage. Contemp Orthoped 19:401, 1989.
42. Mankin HJ: The reaction of articular cartilage to injury and osteoarthritis. Medical progress. N Engl J Med 291:1335, 1974.
43. Weiss C: Ultrastructure characteristics of osteoarthritis. Fed Proc 32:1459, 1973.

CHAPTER 7

The Spastic Hand

UPPER MOTOR NEURON DISEASE

The hand that becomes spastic as a result of a central nervous system impairment such as cerebral palsy or stroke presents specific therapeutic problems. The neocortex involvement in hand function has been thoroughly covered in Chapter 2 of this volume.

Loss of neural control of the intricate mechanisms of hand function is a formidable impairment to the afflicted patient. Evaluation of the components of a spastic upper extremity is reasonably simple, but correction of the deficit with known therapeutic modalities is less rewarding.

Wynn Parry aptly stated the problem of the adult hemiplegic as follows:[1]

> Anything more than a transient hemiplegia results in "permanent" paralysis of the intrinscs (muscles) of the hand. Lumbrical and interrosseous actions hardly ever return. There may be some coarse movement in the thumb, even some opposition, but controlled fine movements are not possible. All that can be expected of a hemiplegic hand is coarse grip and support.

This assertion does not negate treatment efforts nor designate all attempts to restore hand function as useless. It is rather a plea for realistic evaluation of impairment, and of outcomes assessment of proferred treatment regimes in respect to intensity, duration, and emotional and financial expenditure.

Long-term meaningful recovery of function is more feasible in children, as the cortex and neurological synaptic connections are more

256

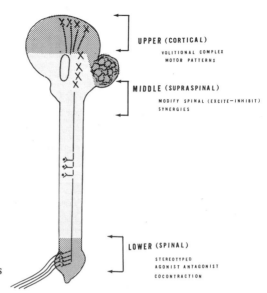

UPPER (CORTICAL)
VOLITIONAL COMPLEX
MOTOR PATTERNS

MIDDLE (SUPRASPINAL)
MODIFY SPINAL (EXCITE—INHIBIT)
SYNERGIES

LOWER (SPINAL)
STEREOTYPED
AGONIST ANTAGONIST
COCONTRACTION

Figure 7–1. Central nervous system.

plastic and malleable. New pathways allegedly can be remodeled, whereas in the adult nervous system retraining is more difficult, longer, and less rewarding.

In the evolution of the central nervous system, higher centers of complex patterns develop to inhibit and modify grosser basic patterns (Fig. 7–1). In cerebrovascular accident this inhibitory modifying contol of gross basic patterns is lost and the latter emerge and predominate. Jackson postulated that the higher centers are cortical regulators that modify the lower basic patterns and gradually develop complex patterns of motor activity.[2]

The cerebral cortex is being studied as to its role in reaching and manual dexterity and in accomplishing desired motor activity. There are several cortical areas with sensorimotor that contribute to the end result.[3-5]

There are also internuncial pools within the subcortal center that must be inhibited to eliminate or modify involuntary reflex activities. Normally these motor patterns are influenced, modified, and inhibited by sensory feedback impulses. It is through these sensory feedback systems that many attempts at rehabilitation are made.

Loss of these central controls results ultimately in spasticity and loss of precise motor activities.

NATURAL HISTORY OF STROKE

The stages of hemiplegia in adult stroke have been well documented by Twitchell:[6]

20 hours:

1. Immediately after hemiplegia there is a total loss of voluntary function and loss or decrease of tendon reflexes.
2. Flaccidity or decrease in resistant to passive movement. Total flaccidity is uncommon.*

48 hours:

3. Deep tendon reflexes increase with possible clonus first noted in finger flexors. There is also noted marked resistance to passive abduction of the upper arm and to extension of the elbow.

3–31 days:

4. Clasp knife phenomenon appears in elbow flexors. Recovery usually (Fig. 7–2) begins in shoulder flexion in the first 6 to 33 days followed by total flexion synergy† spreading distally in the

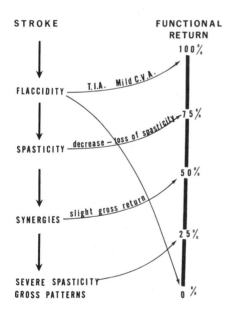

Figure 7–2. Estimate of spontaneous recovery from stroke.

---

*The initial weakness is found in the distal musculature such as the hand intrinsics. Deep tendon reflexes are initially lost, with the onset of hypotonia.

†*Synergy:* combined, coordinated action.

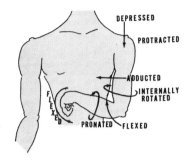

Figure 7–3. Flexor synergy of upper extremity.

extremity. This " total" synergy is not universal, thus recovery does not always follow an identical pattern. With the flexor components of the total synergy spasticity may occur and remain in one component of the upper extremity spastic pattern and not in another.

The synergy pattern that develops in the upper extremity is flexor in type, with flexion of the elbow, adduction of the shoulder, internal rotation of the arm, pronation of the forearm and flexion of the wrist and fingers, thumb in palm (Fig. 7–3).

Loss of "isolated" movements of the fingers, in all skilled motions of the hand, presents a severe functional impairment. The thumb is adducted and opposed into the palm. There is also a loss of wrist and finger extension.

Recovery of voluntary control is usually preceded by diminution of flexor synergy and a decrease of spasticity (Fig. 7–4). These have been staged by Brunnstrom:[7]

Stage I: Flaccidity.
Stage II: Gradual development of spasticity beginning with synergies.
Stage III: Increase in spasticity with some return of voluntary control (if patient is improving).
Stage IV: Decline of spasticity with increasing control of components of the synergy. Recovery may end at this stage with persistence of the remaining synergy component or partial decrease of the total synergy.
Stage V: Synergies no longer control motor acts.
Stage VI: Development of individual joint movement and early coordination.

In patients who will undergo spontaneous motor recovery, 40 percent regain full motion of the arm.[8] Within the first 2 weeks, these

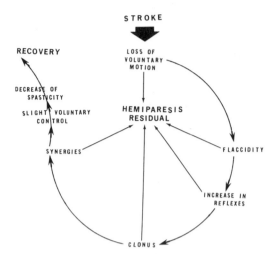

Figure 7–4. Stages of recovery from stroke.

patients show initial return of the shoulder, elbow, and hand motions, all of which show simultaneous recovery during that week. In those that can be expected to fully recover, full motion will usually be noted within 4 weeks and always within the first 3 months. Forty percent regain partial movement with continued improvement up to 7 months. Twenty percent show no return of function.

The site of meaningful recovery in the upper extremity varies. Full return of motion is usually noted in the elbow, less in the hand and "least in the shoulder." Full range of motion of the hand and arm, and also practical function, are usually not regained, as there is often an associated apraxia, dystonia, sensory loss, loss of coordination, perceptual loss, and intellectual impairment.

Carroll claimed that "no return of function within a week indicates that there will not be a return of full 'use' of the extremity."[9] "Use" here implied serviceable function of hand-finger and shoulder activities involving adequate sensation and coordination. Return of meaningful sensation may occur in time,[10] with the prognosis being more guarded when two-point discrimination disturbance persists.

There are numerous factors that influence upper extremity return of function. These must be considered and addressed in considering rehabilitation:

1. Natural sequential return of function independent of treatment modalities.[11]
2. Spasticity — degree and progression.
3. Predominance and persistence of primitive reflex pattern synergies.

4. Apraxia.
5. Contractures.
6. Peripheral sensory deficit (occurs in 80% of stroke cases).
7. Perceptual involvement.[12]
8. Intellectual impairment.
9. Functional loss of the hand because of incompetence of shoulder function.
10. Neurological complication, such as reflex sympathetic dystrophy, causing pain and soft tissue impairment (see Chapter 3).
11. Associated reactions. These are involuntary movements occurring in the paretic extremity in association with movements in other parts of the body. These occur in approximately 80 percent of stroke patients.[13] They may be of no functional significance but they do raise false hopes of improvement.

Functional return 11 to 12 weeks after stroke has been noted.[14] Only 34 percent of patient's could grasp an object with their afflicted hand and none (0%) could perform alternate or repetitive finger movements. Only 9 percent could retrieve an object from the floor, 25 percent turn a door knob, 24 percent grasp a coin, and only 24 percent drop a coin in a slot. All these tested motions required isolated individual finger motions that eluded recovery.

TREATMENT

The position of the patient immediately after onset of hemiplegia is influenced by gravity, as reflexes are lost and the perception of space is impaired. The synergic attitude of the hand is assumed, in which the arm is adducted and internally rotated, the forearm pronated, and fingers, and wrist assume a flexed position. As the patient is unable to overcome these forces, "passive" intervention is required to place the patient in the desired physiologic position (Fig. 7–5). Pillows placed under the arm keep the arm from the body in a 90° abduction and ensure external rotation. The elbow is kept at 90° and the hand is elevated to minimize edema. The wrist is maintained in a slightly extended position with the use of towels or splints. The fingers should be kept slightly extended and the thumb in abduction, yet in a position of slight opposition.

In the acute phase, static splints are indicated, to be replaced by dynamic splints (see Fig. 10–1, static rest splint) as function and or spasticity occurs.

During this flaccid phase, gentle passive range-of-motion exercises

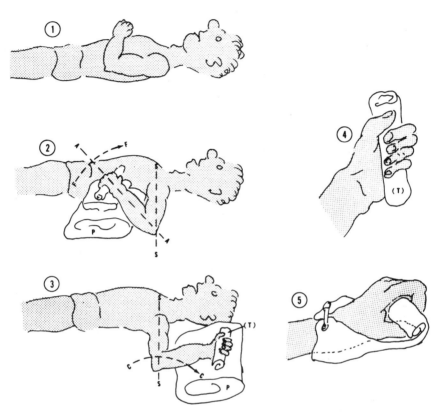

Figure 7–5. Arm, hand, and finger positioning during acute phase of hemiplegia. (1) The usual position of the arm — adducted to the body, elbow flexed, wrist and fingers flexed, and forearm pronated. (2) Pillows (P) are placed to abduct the arm to horizontal position (SS), forearm slightly externally rotated (FF), wrist extended as in 4 or 5. (3) When sufficiently mobile, the arm in the abducted position (SS) is externally rotated (CC) until resting upon the pillow. Wrist and fingers are kept in extension using a rolled face towel (T). (4) Rolled face towel is placed in the hemiplegic hand keeping the fingers slightly extended and the thumb *ab*ducted. (5) A towel folded and pinned as shown can keep the wrist extended and help keep the fingers from a clenched posture.

should be administered several times daily to ensure that the joints are brought to physiologic range of motion. These exercises are to prevent or minimize contracture. They should not be forceful or excessive, nor past the physiological range since proprioception is impaired and the patient unable to inform the therapist or resist the motion, and subluxation of a joint can be easily incurred.

As most activities are assumed by the uninvolved side, the affected side should be involved in all motions as soon as possible. The uninvolved side is usually untrained, having not been the predominant hand; thus; training is necessary. The affected hand should also be involved in assistive activities requiring two hands.

Rehabilitation Potential

There are criteria that should be invoked in determining the rehabilitation potential of the stroke patient and the treatment prognosis.[15] These include acceptance of disability by the patient and the family: bladder control: good visual motor coordination; early return of muscle tone, deep tendon reflexes, and voluntary motor activity; good strength in hand and trunk muscles; and skill in feeding activities.

Most patients make significant gains in a rehabilitation program; therefore a trial period is justified.[16]

Restoration of motor function is obviously the goal of rehabilitation therapy. There are numerous different techniques of physical therapy; all allegedly based on basic neurophysiologic concepts.

Traditional Programs

Traditionally all exercise programs emphasize vigorous range-of-motion exercises to prevent contracture of the affected limb and to assist in retraining of the contralateral, uninvolved limb.[17,18]

Programs Based on Neurophysiologic Concepts

These techniques all attempt to bring the primitive patterns under voluntary control by isolation of specific motions of the patterns being attempted. Most of these programs have several common features:

1. Use of sensory input to facilitate desired or inhibit unwanted motor function.
2. Utilization of the physiologic developmental motor functions.
3. Utilization of involuntary reflex activities to facilitate or inhibit motor activities.
4. Repetition of gained motor activities.
5. Total integration of the body with specific extremity activities.[19]

Most procedures require extensive training and acceptance of the techniques, plus the ability on the part of the patient to undergo the prolonged duration of treatment. Outcomes assessment of functional return often determines whether the financial burden required to continue the treatment can be accepted.

Regaining practical function requires overcoming, to a significant degree, the opposing spasticity and restoring the agonist-antagonist relationship. The use of pathologic reflexes are involved in regaining normal patterns in many of these techniques

Several of the numerous techniques for regaining motor function have survived the years of implementation by occupational and physical therapists.

The Bobath method is based on "release" of the heirarchy of functions of the nervous sytem through sensory input and motor feedback.[20] The patient is urged to accomplish a specific motor activity while the therapist holds the extremity in that precise position. Treatment begins in the supine then side-lying, prone, sitting, kneeling, and finally upright postures. Sensory stimulation is a large component of the technique.

Rood emphasizes cutaneous sensory stimulation to regain the patterns that have been learned during development.[21] These stimulations are brushing, touching, and stroking over precise skin areas. Both agonist and antagonist areas and muscle groups are incorporated.

The Brunnstrom method follows the stages of recovery described by Twitchell. These begin with flaccidity, then spasticity, and are followed by the development of synergies, increased control of synergies, and finally with return of voluntary control.[22] Brunnstrom uses synergies to facilitate rather than suppress unwanted motions. Sensory cutaneous reflex and proprioceptive stimulus techniques are used.[23]

The proprioceptive neuromuscular facilitation (PNF) method originated by Kabat was developed by Knott and Voss.[23] This technique utilizes stretching of basic neuromuscular patterns of the upper extremities with resistance to these patterns that result from the stretching. Patterns allegedly contained in the midbrain are used, as are tonic neck and tonic labyrinthine reflexes. Repetitive responses are prominent.

Slow passive stretching of spastic muscle groups is effective, albeit short-lived and not of prolonged functional value.

Modalities

Cryotherapy. Cryotherapy is effective to temporarily reduce spasticity.[24] While its effect is temporary it allows exercises to be employed during its application. The application of ice to the hand of the hemiplegic is very effective in eliminating and minimizing the ravages of RSD in hemiplegic extremities (Chapter 3). Cold apparently decreases the activity of the muscle spindle and allows elongation of the extrafusal fibers.

Biofeedback. Biofeedback through electromyographic technique has been attempted to regain upper extremity function. Benefit in treatment of shoulder subluxation has been claimed,[25] but practical hand recovery has been less successful.[26,27]

Functional Electrical Stimulation. Although functional electrical stimulation (FES) has been effective in gait training,[28] it has been less valuable in upper extremity retraining, except for some value in wrist function.[29] The intricacies of neuromuscular activities in the hand make FES very difficult to carry out and it is currently inapplicable.

Orthosis

Orthotic devices for the upper extremity in stroke patients are used primarily to prevent contractures. Occasionally they are of value to alleviate pain.[30] They have proven to be effective in affording functional assistance or substituting functions.[31]

Because of the spasticity usually incurred in stroke stimulation, initiating spastic reaction must be avoided. Since volar splints may cause pressure on the palmar muscles and skin and initiate a flexion spasticity, they may need to be avoided or used sparingly. Dorsal splints avoid this cutaneous stimulus and thus are more practical when indicated. A dorsal splint may be used during waking hours and a palmar splint at night.

Medications

Medications to bring about release or diminution of spasticity have been tried with some success.[32] These are predominently dantrolene, baclofen, and diazepam. Phenytoin, chlorpromazine and propranolol, a beta blocker, have some advocates. Their doseage, indications, and contraindications are beyond the scope of this text but are readily available in pertinent references.[32,33]

Surgical Intervention in the Spastic Hand

Surgery on the hand has been performed primarily to correct deformity, relieve pain, and even conceivably to improve function. The procedures to improve function are limited to patients who have reasonably adequate motor function with good sensation but are impaired by contracture or opposing flexor spasticity.[34] Major improvement has been achieved in improving extensor functions of the thumb, wrist, and fingers having overcome the flexor opposition.

There have been criteria imposed upon the selection of patients who may benefit from these surgical procedures.[34] To be a suitable candidate the patient should:

1. Be motivated, be mentally competent and have suffered the stoke at least 9 months ago
2. Have some selective voluntary extension function of the digit being considered for surgical intervention.
3. Should be using that extremity for some functional activities.
4. Should have intact proprioception.
5. Should have two-point discrimination at less than 10 mm distance, and preferably at a 5 mm separation.
6. Should have no joint contracture.

Surgical remedy of contractures presents another challenge.[35] Surgery for contractures in the spastic extremity has usually been relegated to application to a nonfunctional extremity when pain is prominent from the contractures and ADL activities are limited. Approaches to contracture of the shoulder and elbow have been beneficial, and hand contractures less effective.

When joint contractures have been adequately (functionally) managed by passive stretching, flexor tendon lengthening and/or transfers can be considered to correct the deficiency. Finger flexion contractures without wrist limitation can also benefit from tendon lengthening. Extensor tenodesis of the wrist is valuable if improper positions of the wrist add to the improper function of the hand.

Before attempting surgery, a careful functional assessment of the patient and hand must be carried out in light of the above criteria stated.

Pain in the stroke patient's hand needs careful evaluation as to the cause. Spasticity per se is an unusual cause, yet it may compound a pain problem. Central stroke pain is a factor to be considered.[36] Attempted movement of a contracted joint may elicit pain. Degenerative articular changes certainly can contribute to pain. Reflex sympathetic dystrophy (RSD) is also a contributor to pain and has been addressed in Chapter 3.

Finding the cause (mechanism) of pain indicates the intervention that should be attempted, that is, therapeutic modalities, medications, and/or surgery.

Training in Activities of Daily Living

Since recovery of individual motor control and coordination remain limited in stroke patients, self-care also remains limited, and training in activities of daily living (ADL) remains desirable. Most ADL activities are accomplished by the use of the other hand, using the impaired hand as an assist,[36] and to do this training is needed.

REFERENCES

1. Wynn Parry CB: Rehabilitation of the Hand. Butterworths, London, 1966, pp 216–217.
2. Jackson JH: On some implications of dissolution of the nervous system. Med Press Circ 2:411, 1882.
3. Kalaska JF, Crammond DJ: Cerebral cortical mechanisms of reaching movements. Science 255: 1517–1523, 1992.
4. Shatz CJ: Dividing up the neocortex. Science 258: 237–238, 1992.
5. Kandel ER, Hawkins RD: The biological basis of learning and individuality. Sci Am 79–88, 1992.
6. Twitchell TE: The restoration of motor function following hemiplegia. Brain 74:443, 1951.
7. Brunnstrom S: Movement Therapy in Hemiplegia: A Neurophysiological Approach. Harper & Row, New York, 1970.
8. Bard G. Hirschberg G: Recovery of voluntary motion in upper extremity following hemiplegia. Arch Phys Med Rehab 45:567, 1965.
9. Carroll D: Hand function in hemiplegia. J Chronic Dis 18:493, 1965.
10. Van Buskirk C, Webster D: Prognostic value of sensory deficit in rehabilitation of hemiplegia. Neurology 5:407, 1955.
11. Pesyczynski ZM: The status of research on recovery of function in hemiplegia. Presented at Fifteenth Scientific Session of the French Society of Prevention and Social Medicine, Paris, Sept 1967.
12. Birch HD, Proctor F, Bortner M, et al,: Perception in hemiplegia. Judgement of vertical and horizontal by hemiplegic patients. Arch Phys Med 41:19, 1960.
13. Anderson EK: Sensory impairment in hemiplegia. Arch Phys Med Rehabil 52:293–297, 1971.
14. Shah SK, Corones J: Volition following hemiplegia. Arch Phys Med Rehabil 61:423–428, 1980.
15. Gersten JW: Rehabilitation potential. In: Licht S (ed.): Stroke and Its Rehabilitation. Elizabeth Licht, New Haven, Conn., 1975, pp 435–471.
16. Lieberman JS: Hemiplegia: Rehabilitation of the upper extremity. In Kaplan PE, Cerullo LJ (eds.): Stroke Rehabilitation. Butterworths, MA, 1986, pp 95–117.
17. Westcott EJ: Traditional exercise regimens for the hemiplegic patient. Am J Phys Med 46:1012–1023, 1967.
18. Swenson JR: Therapeutic exercises in hemiplegia. In Basmajian JV (ed): Therapeutic Exercise, ed.3. Williams & Wilkins, Baltimore, 1978, pp 325–348.
19. Flanagan EM: Methods of facilitation and inhibition of motor activity. Am J Phys Med 46:1006–1011, 1967.

20. Bobath B: Adult Hemiplegia: Evaluation and Treatment. William Heinemann, London, 1970.
21. Rood M: Neurophysiological reactions as a basis for physical therapy. Phys Ther Rev 34:444, 1954.
22. Brunnstrom SS: Movement therapy in hemiplegia: a neurophysiological approach. Harper & Row, New York, 1970.
23. Knott M, Voss DE: Proprioceptive Neuromuscular Facilitation, ed 2. Harper & Row, New York, 1968.
24. Michlovitz SL: Cryotherapy: The use of cold as a therapeutic agent. In Michlovitz SL (ed): Thermal Agents in Rehabilitation, ed 2. FA Davis, Philadelphia, 1990, pp 63–87.
25. Basmajian JV: Biofeedback in therapeutic exercise. In Basmajian JV (ed.): Therapeutic Exercise, 3rd ed. Williams & Wilkins, Baltimore, 1978, pp 220–227.
26. Basmajian JV, Gowland C, Brandstater ME, Swanson L, Trotter J: EMG feedback treatment of upper limb in hemiplegic stroke patients: a pilot study. Arch Phys Med Rehabil 63:613–616, 1982.
27. Bowman BR, Baker LL, Waters RL: Positional feedback and electrical stimulation: an automated treatment for the hemiplegic wrist. Arch Phys Med Rehabil 60:497–502, 1979.
28. Vodovnik L, Kralj A, Stanic U, Acimovic R, Gros N: Recent applications of functional electrical stimulation to stroke patients in Ljubljana. Clin Orthop 131:64–70, 1978.
29. Merletti R, Acrimovic R, Grobelnik S, Cvilak G: Electrophysiological orthosis for the upper extremity in hemiplegia: feasibility study. Arch Phys Med Rehabil 56:507–513, 1975.
30. McCollough NC: Orthotic management in adult hemiplegia. Clin Orthop 131–146, 1978.
31. Wilson D, Caldwell CB: Central control insufficiency, III: disturbed motor control and sensation: a treatment approach emphasizing upper extremity orthosis. Phys Ther 58:313–320, 1978.
32. Young RR, Delwaide PJ: Drug therapy: spasticity (first of two parts). N Engl J Med 304:28–33, 1981.
33. Young RR, Delwaide PJ: Drug therapy: spasticity (second of two parts). N Engl J Med 304:96–99, 1981.
34. Waters RL: Upper extremity surgery in stroke patients. Clin Orthop 131:30–37, 1978.
35. Treanor WJ: Improvement of function in hemiplegia after stroke surgery. Scand J Rehabil Med 13:123–135, 1981.
36. Cailliet R: Pain: Mechanisms and Management. FA Davis, Philadelphia, 1993.
37. Boivie J, Leijon G: Clinical findings in patients with central stroke pain, In Casey KL (ed): Pain and Central Nervous System Disease: The Central Pain Syndromes, Raven Press, New York, 1991, pp 65–76.
38. Kamenetz L: Occupational therapy for the stroke patient. In Licht S (ed.): Stroke and its Rehabilitation. Elizabeth Licht, New Haven, Conn., 1975, pp 347–379.

CHAPTER 8

Thermal and Electrical Burns of the Hand

The hand is covered by skin (Fig. 8–1) which has two major layers: the epidermis and the dermis. The outermost layer of the epidermis, called the "stratum corneum," is a nonvascular stratified epithelium containing fibrils and fat globules. With ample hydration the long hydrocarbon chains containing fat globules are suspended in water, allowing them to remain separated and flexible. Dehydration causes these fibrils to adhere to and lose their flexibility.

The dermis is a "feltwork" of bundles of white fibers and elastic fibers. Within it are located blood vessels, nerve endings, hair follicles, and sweat glands. The major blood vessels run within the subcutaneous tissues and small branches supply the dermis.

The underlying fascia consists of bundles of white collagenous fibers, that form a webbing, some elastin fibers and filled with tissue fluid. The deep fascia covers muscles, tendons, and bone. Burns that affect the hands initially injure the skin in any or all of its layers.

In recent years the mortality and morbidity of hand burns has diminished because of advances in wound care, intense care of the burned hand, and attention to nutritional support.[1] The hand is burned in more than 89 percent of patients admitted to burn units.[2]

Appropriate initial management of the burned hand is critical in assuring ultimate functional recovery. Several principles must be considered:

1. Edema prevention.
2. Avoidance of prolonged immobilization.
3. Proper positioning.

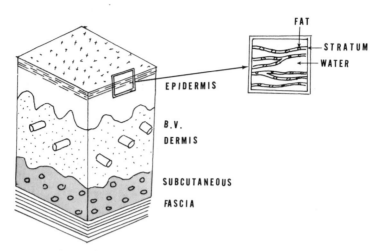

Figure 8–1. Skin (schematic). A cube of skin is depicted with all layers indicated. The square in the upper right is an enlargement of the epidermis. The strata contains fibrilla which contain fat globules in a matrix of water. The small blood vessels (**BV**) are contained within the dermis layer.

4. Prevention of infection.
5. Preservation of the remaining viable tissue.

CLASSIFICATIONS OF BURNS

The degree of the burn must be ascertained, since it dictates the treatment and underlies the prognostic factors (Table 8–1).

The appearance of the burn gives an indication of the severity but not always an accurate evaluation of the degree. A first degree burn is painful with demonstrable erythema and early edema of varying degree. A second degree burn is either superficial or deep, it involves the

Table 8–1 CLASSIFICATION OF BURNS

Degree	*Depth*	*Appearance*
First	Epidermis	Erythema
Second	Superficial and deep dermis	Blistering
Third	Full-thickness skin loss	Leathery blanched appearance
Fourth	Full-thickness loss with damage of underlying muscle, tendon, and bone	Nonviable structures visible

epidermis and varying degrees of dermis. It too is painful and blanches under pressure, and usually presents with blistering. A third degree burn presents with full-thickness loss of skin and leaves an anesthetic surface having leathery appearance. In a fourth degree burn, all underlying tissues are visible.

The cause of the burn is an indicator of severity. Wet heat penetrates more deeply than does dry heat and often causes a third degree burn. An electric burn produces a heat five times the intensity of a thermal burn and also causes third degree burns. Chemical burns usually are second degree.

Determination of the local circulation helps determine whether a burn is a second or third degree burn. A first or second degree burn is indicated when pressure applied with a sterile hemostat causes blanching followed by reddening upon release. If the skin does not blanch it is probably a third degree burn. These do not redden upon release of the pressure.

Third degree burns form carbon monoxide within the burn site. The carbon monoxide fixes the hemoglobin, creating a brilliant red hue to the area. This color does not blanch upon pressure and is a reliable diagnostic sign determining degree.

With a second degree burn the skin is usually thicker than normal upon palpation, whereas in a third degree burn the skin is thinner. This relative thickness is manually determined by moving a sterile gloved finger along the adjacent skin. Upon reaching the burned skin region an "elevation" implies a second degree burn, whereas a " depression" suggests a third degree burn. Loss of sensation is not an indication of degree, as all burns display a degree of sensory loss.

MANAGEMENT

When the hand is burned to a severe degree almost *all* the hand is affected. It is impossible to generalize regarding the care of the burned hand, as care depends on the severity of the burn, the precise location(s), the tissue(s) involved, the circulation. Immediate care should evolve into "early" rehabilitation as maintenance of function is paramount.

Management of the acute phase of a hand burn consists of pain control, wound healing, maintainance of range of motion, and prevention of infection. As a general rule, an exercise program is initiated within 48 to 72 hours and is carried out several times a day. Nonburned portions of the extremities are also included in the exercise program.

For minor burns, wound care should consist of cleansing with a mild soap, debridement of ruptured blisters, and dressing with nonadherent gauze. The involved aspect of the hand should be splinted. Topical antibiotics are reserved for the more severely burned hand.

The antibiotics currently advocated are the broad spectrum topical agents silver sulfadiazine and mafenide acetate. The former is broad spectrum painless upon application. The latter penetrates the burn eschar and is useful in electric burns.

For superficial secondary burns, topical antibiotic applications usually result in spontaneous healing with good function. Use of antibiotic is usually preceded by cleansing the burn area with a mild nonirritating soap to remove film, exudate, and previous applications of topical agents. The best cleansing agent is copious amounts of water. The area then should be covered by a dry sterile mesh dressing that stimulates the growth of granulation tissue. A fine mesh dressing helps flatten the areas of new granulation tissue. The dressings are applied wet with sterile water and allowed to dry.

Blisters that are intact are sterile and should be left alone until they reabsorb. Once ruptured they are a focus of infection and the wrinkled skin should be removed.

A debrided second degree burn usually heals with external exposure. A blood clot usually forms that seals the denuded area. After 7 to 10 days, if there is inadequate healing, an "artificial" clot can be initiated. Painting the area with mercurochrome may hasten drying and crusting, as can the application of a sterile dry mesh gauze. As infection is the greatest fear any application MUST be done with complete asepsis: sterile equipment, gloves, mask, and so on.

In deep secondary burns, removal of burned tissue down to a bleeding base and subsequent skin grafting is usually indicated.

In third degree burns, early excision of burned tissue and grafting is desired in an otherwise acceptable patient.

As the majority of upper extremity burns are only a part of a larger burn injury the total patient must be considered. Initial treatment includes preservation of the circulation by early escharotomy and/or fasciotomy as needed, early wound coverage, early range of motion actively and passively, elevation to prevent or relieve edema, proper splinting to avoid joint contracture, and wound sepsis control by topical antibiotics.

Edema is an undesirable sequela of burns and must be actively combatted. The hand must be kept elevated as often and as long as possible. If the patient is otherwise incapacitated and unable to actively elevate the hand, it maybe so elevated by the application of a Fiberglas splint enclosed in a stockinet (Fig. 8–2).

A circumferential burn combined with wound edema can lead to a compartment syndrome. Since many of the hand muscles are in the forearm these compartment syndromes must be addressed early.

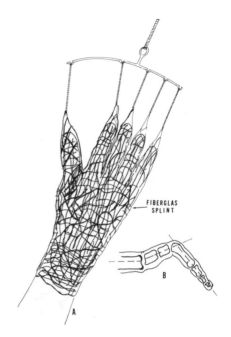

Figure 8-2. Fiberglas splint over stockinet base (A). This splint holds the hand with the wrist in slight extension. The metacarpal joints are in slight flexion and the interphalangeal joints are in extension (B). The hand can be held elevated by an overhead traction.

Compartment Syndrome

Compartment syndrome is a serious complication of any trauma to the extremity and is particularly so in burns. An increase in intracompartmental tissue pressure causes increased venous pressure, decrease in local blood flow, and a lowering of the arteriovenous gradient.

Tension within the extremity with pain and upon passive stretching is an early indication of this condition, as is paresthesia *in spite of intact pulses*. The Doppler sign test is often administered but unfortunately is not an assurance of adequate perfusion. Insertion of a Wick catheter[3] is more accurate and often indicates the need for surgical decompression.

Determining tissue pressures is helpful in monitoring the intracompartmental pressures, but an understanding of the pathophysiology of the compartment syndrome determination of the mean arterial pressures as well as compartmental pressures is valuable.[4] In addition to increased venous pressure there may be an actual collapse of arterial blood vessels with cessation of blood flow.[5] There is currently a plea for monitoring mean arterial pressure within the compartment as well as compartment pressure itself.[5]

Surgical decompression should begin on unburned skin proximal to the burn on both the radial and ulnar borders of the arm, taking care to avoid the peripheral nerves. This escharotomy should extend to the hand and the wrist and, when indicated, even to the midaxial lines of the digits. Decompression of the dorsal interosseous muscles should also be considered.

Splints

Applications of thermoplastic splints to avoid deformity should be initiated early (Fig. 8–3). They are molded of isoprene plastic and applied directly to the part ensuring maximum contact with the fibrous bands of the scar. This produces an unyielding pressure upon the scar that gradually softens and remodels it in the desired position. The joints are also maintained in a functional position. This splint can be molded either on the palmar or volar aspect of the hand, depending on the intensity and region of maximum scarring. If both surfaces of the hand are burned, a volar and dorsal splint may be combined.

Serial splints can be used to correct a contracture. Periodic examination of the hand indictates the degree of change desired. A functional splint using rubber bands can also be used to increase flexibility of scar (see Chapter 10).

Before applying corrective splints several questions should be posed:

1. Will the newly healed skin tolerate the stress and the compression?

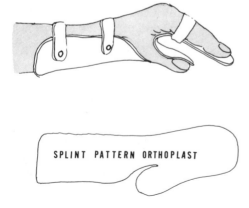

SPLINT PATTERN ORTHOPLAST

Figure 8–3. Isoplast isoprene splint. Models are made in several-size patterns for immediate application. The plastic is heated by hot water or heat gun, then cut and molded easily to the patient's hand. (Adapted from Willis B: The use of orthoplast isoprene splints in the treatment of the acutely burned child. Am J Occup Ther 23:57, 1969.)

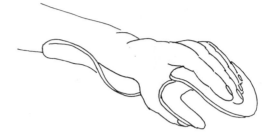

Figure 8-4. Volar splint. In a burned hand a volar slab splint may be applied directly to the skin contour.

2. Will the scar best be treated by constant pressure or by dynamic stretching?[7]
3. Will the patient tolerate the appliance in regard to pain, discomfort, or cosmetic appearance?
4. Can the splint be accepted for the duration required?

The hand should be placed and mantained in a position of 10° to 20° wrist dorsal flexion, thumb in palmar abduction, and the metacarpophalangeal joints in 60° to 80° flexion (Fig. 8-4). When the wrist is slightly flexed it remains functional and permits functional digit (Fig. 8-5) motion. It is not possible to depict every possible splint, as every burn problem presents a different challenge.[8]

The metacarpophalangeal joints are frequently involved in burns of the hand and require special attention. These joints especially tend to contract and usually (in dorsal burns) do so in extension. Any splinting that includes the metacarpophalangeal joint should extend distally to assure flexion of that (those) joints.[9]

With the metacarophalangeal joints flexed the thumb web may permit abduction but restrict extension; therefore the thumb must be passively stretched (extended) frequently. If the thumb has also been burned it should also be included in the splint so that it remains constantly in a stretched position. If the thumb has been so severely burned as to indicate ultimate contracture it should be maintained in a flexed opposed position by either static or kinetic splints.

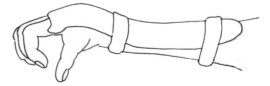

Figure 8-5. Dorsal splint. In a burned hand a dorsal slab splint may be applied directly to the skin contour.

Maintaining Flexibility

Burn scars tend to contract and thicken causing the skin to thicken and the underlying joints to contract. Both skin and joints need attention.

The hand, wrist and fingers must be splinted into a functional position and must be kept as mobile as possible by active-passive exercises.

Gentle sustained stretching lengthens the bands of scar tissue and in turn increases the joint range of motion. Massage after a local paraffin application maintains skin flexibility.

Paraffin has proven to be an effective method of applying heat and skin lubrication. It should be considered only after the skin is physiologically acceptable and not in the blister stage. It will not be accepted if the skin is sensitive to local temperatures of 37°C to 38°C, the temperature of the usual liquid paraffin treatment.

Paraffin has a melting point of 34°C. It is mixed with heavy-duty mineral oil in a ratio of 75 grams of oil to 450 grams paraffin. Once the two substances are dissolved the temperature is reduced to 33°C or slightly less. The hand is immersed in the solution eight to ten times each applying a coat. While being immersed the hand should be actively flexed and extended.

Deep massage involving the subcutaneous tissues must avoid friction of the superficial layers, which can cause blistering. Gentle local heat enhances lubrication and flexibility of the skin and subcutaneous tissue. It also diminishes pain.[6]

Grafts

In the severely burned hand the tissue is debrided and grafting is indicated. The timing of grafting remains unresolved. It is obvious that the sooner the burn wound is healed the less chance there is for subsequent contracture. There is therefore a current tendency to excise burns at the time of injury with immediate split-thickness skin grafting. Earlier functional healing has been claimed from early surgical intervention.[10]

The techniques and types of grafts are beyond the purview of this text, but postoperative care requires active attention to the flexibility of the grafted tissues and the underlying joints of the hand.

Postoperatively, meticulous care must be exercised with regard to wound care, splinting, local treatment, and the precise types of exercises.[11]

REFERENCES

1. Demling RH: Burn. N Engl J Med 313:1389, 1985.
2. Salisbury RE, Dingeldein GP: The burned hand and upper extremity. In Green DP: Operative Hand Surgery, ed 2, Vol 3, Churchill Livingstone, New York, 1988, p 2135.
3. Mubarak SJ, Hargens AR, Owen CA, et al.: The Wick catheter technique for measure of intramuscular pressure. J Bone Joint Surg (Am) 58A:1016, 1976.
4. Mabee JR, Bostwick TL: Pathophysiology and mechanisms of compartment syndrome. Orthop Rev 175–181, 1993.
5. Ashton H: The effect of increased tissue pressure on blood flow. Clin Orthop 113:15–26, 1975.
6. Boswick JA: Rehabilitation of the burned hand. Clin Orthop 104:162, 1974.
7. Koepke GH, Feallock B, Feller I: Splinting of the severely burned hand. Am J Occup Ther 17:147. 1963.
8. Salisbury RE, Palm L, Dynamic splinting for dorsal burns of the hand. Plast Reconstr Surg 51:226, 1973.
9. Schultz-Johnson K: Splinting — a problem-solving approach. In Stanley BG, Tribuzi SM (eds): Concepts in Hand Rehabilitation. FA Davis, Philadelphia, 1992, pp. 238–271.
10. Ross WPD: The treatment of recent burns of the hand. Br J Plast Surg 2:233–253, 1949–1950.
11. Salisbury RE, Wright P: Evaluation of early excision of dorsal burns on the hand. Plast Reconstr Surg 69:670,1982.

CHAPTER 9

Hand Infections

In a treatise published 50 years ago the statement was made that "In almost all cases of serious infection the difficulty is to make the correct diagnosis both as the nature of the infection and the position of the pus."[1] This statement was specifically directed to the hand where infections are of particularly prominent concern.

The first stage in the treatment of hand infections is an accurate and prompt diagnosis regarding the microorganism, the anatomy of the infected site, and the natural course of the infection.

Infections must be classified as to whether they are superficial, subcutaneous, fascial, synovial, bony or compartmental. Compartmental infections pose the greatest concern as they may be directly introduced by trauma or penetration (these are the most prevalent), or they may have entered hematogenously.

MICROBIOLOGY

The most prominent bacterial pathogens are *Staphylococcus aureus*, *Streptococcus* spp., or coliform bacteria. Anaerobic bacteria can also be introduced via penetrating injuries.

Streptococcal infections usually evolve rapidly within 24 to 48 hours and develop into cellulitis. Staphyloccocal infections tend to be superficial, evolving within 3 to 6 days. Chronic infections often include fungi or atypical mycobacteria. Accurate diagnosis requires culture and determination of sensitivity to specific antibiotics.

Preliminary treatment, besides giving local attention to the infected area and tissue, addresses the nature of the specific pathogen.[2] Antibiotic administration may be oral, intramuscular, or even intravenous,

278

depending on the symptomatology and the severity of the infection. The general health status of the host (patient) must be considered, for example the concurrent existence of diabetes or immunodeficiency illnesses.

LOCAL TREATMENT

Local treatment must address the general principles of:

1. Local rest.
2. Immobilization.
3. Edema prevention by elevation.
4. Local heat(advocated by many).
5. Drainage of closed spaces and/or debridement of infected tissues.

Local treatment is started early when pain, erythema, and swelling have begun to subside as a result of antibiotic treatment. The concept that if the infection is not responding within 24 to 48 hours of initial treatment the diagnosis must be questioned and reevaluated has proven to be sound.[3]

Operative drainage is specifically directed to the exact site of the infection and implies accurate understanding of the structures of the involved compartments.

FELON

A pyogenic infection in the terminal pulp space is called a *felon* (Fig. 9–1). Between the bone and the skin the pulp contains numerous (15–20) vertical septa running from the periosteum to the skin, these form compartments. The small nerves and blood vessels coursing through these compartments supply the fingertips.

Once the infection spreads into these compartments there is a painful swelling that occludes the circulation. Ultimately the enclosed bone can undergo necrosis. Thus release of the pressure is considered an emergency.

Usually there is a history of a penetrating injury. The abcess forms centrally in the pulp space and spreads towards the periosteum and the skin. Swelling usually does not extend proximal to the distal interphalangeal joint.

With respect to the configuration of the compartment, any incision can be effective for drainage if the incision is "across" the columns. Due to the sensitivity of the tactile pad surfaces any incision must be made so

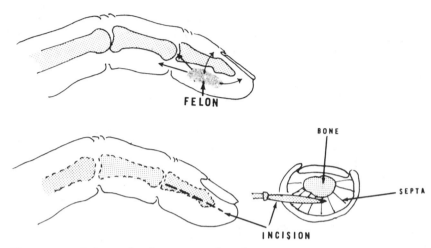

Figure 9–1. Felon, pulp abscess. A pulp infection may spread in the direction shown by the arrows—to the tip, to the dorsum, or retrograde into the distal joint or the flexor tendon sheath. The pulp is divided into compartments by vertical septa. Incision for a felon must cut across these septa and be near the nail to avoid later scarring of the sensitive tactile surface.

as to avoid scarring on the volar surface. Circumferential incisions are to be avoided as they may compromise the blood supply to the distal phalanx. A high lateral incision on the side of maximal tenderness is recommended (see Fig. 9–1).

If the infection has invaded the bone the sequestrum must be excised or it will remain as a focus of infection.

Management after early recognition of the felon therefore demands appropriate antibiotics, adequate incision, and removal of the sequestrum.

PARONYCHIA

The perionychium includes the nail, nail matirx, and the eponychial and paranychial folds. Penetration of the infecting bacteria under the eponychium at the periphery of the nail produces the infection termed *paronychium.* Of the numerous causes, the most common are nail biting, manicures, and hang nails.[4]

Initially there is redness, pain, and swelling that (Fig. 9–2) elevates the skin fold over the base of the nail. The infection tends to spread proximally underneath the nail margin to involve the nail bed.

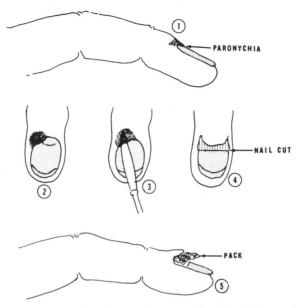

Figure 9–2. Paronychia. This infection begins at the base of the nail (1) and (2). If found early, it may be treated by elevating the overhanging skin by a sharp probe (3) and releasing the pus. If infection is too severe, the nail may be cut (4); the proximal nail is removed exposing the bed, and elevating and packing under the overhanging skin (5) are done.

The most common bacterium in acute paroncyhia is *Staphylococcus aureus.*[5]

If the diagnosis is made before the pus accumulates, oral antibiotics may be curative. Once there is a fluctuant accumulation of pus, drainage is necessary (see Fig. 9–2). If the pus does not extend beneath the nail, drainage is possible by lifting the eponychium of the nail by a blunt probe. After exposure a small piece of mesh gauze is left in the opening.

If the collection extends beneath the nail a longitudinal section of the nail is removed (Fig. 9–3). The eponychium may be incised. If the paronychium extends around the dorsal nail bed, the proximal third of the nail may be removed. In any incision, a small piece of mesh gauze may be left in place to insure total drainage. Appropriate oral antibiotics accompany any incision and drainage.

Chronic paronychia always suggests the possibility of atypical mycobacteria and/or fungi.[6] This occurs mostly in people exposed to constant moisture. Surgical drainage is effective. In some cases this may extend to removing the nail to expose the palmar floor of the nail, followed by administration of topical antifungal agents.

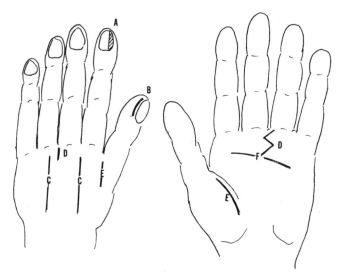

Figure 9-3. Sites of incision for drainage of hand infections. The sites of incision are indicated by the precise infection site. As a rule, dorsal incisions are longitudinal and palmar incisions conform to the lines of cleavage. (A) Paronychia, (B) felon, (C) dorsal space, (D) web space, (E) the thenar space (both palmar and dorsal), and (F) midpalmar space.

SYNOVIAL SPACE INFECTIONS

Bacterial infection of the closed synovial sheaths of the flexor tendons causes an acute flexor tenosynovitis. The flexor tendon sheath has a visceral layer adhering to the tendon that extends to the midpalmar crease.[7] There are two palmar bursae that surround the superficial and deep flexor tendons. They extend proximal to the transverse carpal ligament.[7] In 80 percent of the population these bursae communicate.

Usually this infection is the result of a penetrating injury. The cardinal symptoms (of acute flexor tenosynovitis) are:[1]

1. Excessive tenderness over the course of the tendon sheath.
2. Symmetrical enlargement of the whole finger.
3. Excruciating pain on passive extension of the finger. This is considered the cardinal symptom.[7]
4. The finger usually assumes a flexed position at rest.

Due to the constricted area within the sheath there is propensity to early tendon necrosis which demands early release of the tension. In early cases, or when the diagnosis is not yet clear, elevation, splinting to immobilize, and intravenous antibiotics are indicated.

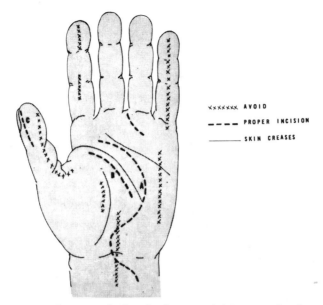

xxxxxx AVOID

- - - - PROPER INCISION

_____ SKIN CREASES

Figure 9–4. Site of incision for hand infections. (A) Incision for drainage of the palmar space between the median and ulnar nerves. The incision curves across the wrist crease to avoid contracture. (B) The incision for draining the thenar space parallels the thenar crease. (C) The incision for drainage of felon transects fascial planes and avoids tactile surfaces. Cutting should be avoided *across* creases, over nerves and blood vessels, and through tactile surfaces.

If there is not improvement within 24 hours incision and drainage is indicated.[8] The zigzag incision to be used is depicted in Fig. 9–4. An irrigation catheter is passed in a retrograde direction through the sheath. The area is then irrigated with copious fluid while the hand is elevated and antibiotics are instilled intravenously. Once the catheter can be removed, active and passive exercises must be initiated.

DEEP PALMAR FASCIAL SPACES

The deep fascial spaces include the dorsal subaponeurotic space, the subfascial web space, the midpalmar space, and the thenar space. These are vulnerable in deep penetrating traumata or hematogenous spread.

The dorsal subaponeurotic space lies beneath the extensor tendons on the dorsum of the hand. Infection of the space presents as a swelling and erythema of the hand. It resembles a dorsal subcutaneous infection and may be difficult to specifically diagnose.[9] If there is any question as to the depth of the infection, incision and drainage are indicated.

The subfascial space commonly results from an infected blister as the skin is adherent to the underlying fascia, which is contiguous with the dorsal subcutaneous spaces of the digits. Incision and drainage are indicated.

The thenar space is contained within a vertical septum between the third metacarpal and middle finger profundus ulnarly, and the lateral edge of the adductor pollicis radially.[1] The adductor pollicis forms the dorsal roof of the compartment. Acute infection presents with swelling and tension of the thenar eminence. The thumb is held in abduction, and passive adduction causes extreme discomfort. The examination reveals a "dumbell" or "pantaloon" appearance of the hand in the region of the first dorsal interosseous muscle.

The midpalmar space is bordered radially by the septum between the third metacarpal and the sheath of the middle finger profundus tendon, and ulnarly by the hypothenar muscles. The dorsal roof is formed by the fascia over the second and third palmar interossei and the third and fourth metacarpals. The compartment is deep to the flexor tendons.

In infection within this compartment the normal transverse palmar arch is lost so that the palm appears convex and tender.

Incision into the palmar area of the hand must avoid cutting the neurovascular bundles, hence the incisions sites indicated in Fig. 9–4. Palmar incisions should parallel the thenar creases, and dorsal incisions should extend along the radial border of the first dorsal interosseous muscle.

Operative drainage requires wide exposure, and the wound must be left open, with the hand splinted in a physiologic position. A bloodless field, achieved by wrapping the entire extremity is elastic dressing and applying a blood pressure cuff over 250 mm Hg, gives excellent exposure. The use of antibiotics of specific to the injection is mandatory.

SEPTIC ARTHRITIS

Any joint of the hand can undergo septic arthritis. Usually these infections are due to a direct penetrating wound that causes a contiguous infection, but they may be hematogenous. Patients with rheumatoid arthritis are particularly vulnerable, as their immune responses are deficient. The enzymes and toxins released by the bacteria can degrade the cartilage.[10] Early drainage (within 16 hours) of a septic hand minimizes this possibility and ensures recovery.[11]

An infected joint becomes warm, swollen, red, tender, and painful upon movement. Careful palpation of the area determines whether the pain is from the tendon or the joint.[12]

A suspected joint should be aspirated under sterile conditions and the fluid should be examined by culture and under the microscope. A purulent fluid is cloudy in appearance and has over 50,000 white cells per cubic millimeter.

Infected joints present an emergency demanding drainage and debridement at the site of aspiration. The incision depends upon the site and the specific joint involved, always bearing in mind the structure and function of the overlying soft tissues. Insertion of a catheter depends upon the judgement of the surgeon once the nature of the organism and the extent of the infection have been determined.

Once the infection is under control, usually in 3 to 6 days, active hand therapy should be instituted to regain function. Significant articular erosion from the infection may mandate ultimate arthroplasty, amputation, or fusion.[13]

BITES TO THE HAND

Bites to the hand are usually upon the dorsum of the clenched fist and involve the skin, subcutaneous tissue, the tendon sheaths, and even the periarticular soft tissue. The offending bacteria are those within the saliva of the biter and should be precisely identified and urgently treated. Early debridement and repair of the damaged tissues must be addressed.

FUNGAL INFECTIONS

Fungal infections should be considered in all chronic skin and fingernail lesions. Microscopic examination and culture reveal the precise organism and treatment with an appropriate fungicide can be initiated.[14]

REFERENCES

1. Kanavel AB: Infections of the Hand. Lea & Febiger Philadelphia, 1939, pp 17–410.
2. Levy CS: Treating infections of the hand: identifying the organism and choosing the antibiotic. In Greene WB (ed): Instructional Course Lectures, Vol 39. AAOS, Park Ridge, 1990, pp 533–537.
3. Hausman MR, Lisser SP: Hand Infections In Common Hand Problems. Orthop Clin North Am 23:171–185, 1992.
4. Stern PJ: Selected acute infections. In Greene WB (ed): Instructional Course Lectures, Vol 39. AAOS, Park Ridge, 1990, pp 539–546.
5. Canales FL, Newmeyer WL Kilgore ES: The treatment of felons and paronychias. Hand Clin 5:553–559, 1989.

6. Barlow AJ, Chattaway FW, Holgate MC, et al.: Chronic paronychia. Br J Dermatol 82:448–453, 1970.
7. Neviaser RJ: Tenosynovitis. Hand Clin 5:525–531, 1989.
8. Neviaser RJ: Infections. In Greene DP (ed): Operative Hand Surgery. Churchill Livingstone, New York, 1988, pp 1027–1047.
9. Burkhalter WE: Deep space infections. Hand Clin 5:553–559, 1989.
10. Petty WE, Fajgenbaum MC: Infection of synovial joints. In Evarts C (ed): Surgery of the Musculoskeletal System. Churchill Livingstone, New York, 1983, pp 4399–4427.
11. Rashkoff ES, Burkhalter WE, Mann RJ: Septic arthritis of the wrist. J Bone Joint Surg (Am) 65A:824–828, 1983.
12. Schurman DJ, Smith RL: Surgical approach to the management of septic arthritis. Orthop Rev 16:241, 1987.
13. Moore MM, Hixson ML, Strickland JW: Infected arthroplasties in the hand and wrist. In Evarts C (ed): Surgery of the Musculoskeletal System. Churchill Livingstone, New York, 1983, 4515–4524.
14. Hitchcock TF, Amadio PC: Fungal infections. Hand Clin 5:599–611, 1989.

CHAPTER 10

Splinting the Hand

TYPES OF SPLINTS

Proper splinting of the hand demands thorough evaluation of impaired hand function and determining precisely what is required of the splint.

The following questions need to be asked and answered:[1]

1. What problems exist in the hand?
2. Which of these problems are amendable to splinting?
3. Which splinting approach will enhance the patient's immediate and ultimate function?
4. How many joints need be included?
5. How much surface contact is needed and/or accepted by the condition?
6. Which material is optimum for proper construction and utilization?
7. How will the splint be maintained on the hand?
8. What forces need to be implemented by the splint?
9. How often need the splint be applied and for how long?
10. Can the splint be applied by the patient without assistance?
11. How will the patient interact with the splint?

Splints can be classified as static, semistatic, semidynamic, or dynamic. These basic types fulfill the following functions:

1. Stabilize joints in a desired position, to rest the joint, tendons, ligaments, and muscles.
2. Maintains a certain bone alignment. Prevent deformity.
3. Prevents contracture of the associated soft tissues.
4. Prevents unwanted motion.

5. Gradually stretches contracture to increase joint motion.
6. Substitutes lost muscle action.
7. Maintains gains that have been achieved by other modalities.
8. Relieves pain.

A splint prescription must therefore indicate the:

1. Anatomical and physiological "problem."
2. The type of splint.
3. Goal of splinting.
4. Frequency and duration of splinting.

Static Splints

A static splint prevents motion and thus rests the part immobilized. It should immobilize "only" the joint intended and thus should be molded according to the contours of the part included and cause no undue or unacceptable pressure. The duration of splinting, as well as the type, should be carefully monitored, as any splinting can result in disuse atrophy, weakness, stiffness, and dependency. It can be stated that *a static splint should never be used if a dynamic or semidynamic performs the same intent.*

A resting (static) splint should have smooth margins and surfaces and be molded accurately to the contour of the extremity to avoid unwanted pressures upon bony prominences or nerve and/or vascular areas.

Circular casts should be avoided or at least minimized as they may become constrictive. If such a cast appears indicated it is best applied as two half slabs held by an elastic binding. A full circular cast should be bivalved as soon as possible.

Semidynamic Splints

This type of splint permits "no" motion but positions the parts being splinted to perform at their optimum. By definition, a semidynamic splint does not use external power sources such as rubber bands or springs. An example of this type of splint is an immobilizer of the thumb that prevents motion in abduction-opposition position yet allows all other motions at that joint and the distal joint to function.

Dynamic Splints

A dynamic splint is also termed a functional or kinetic splint in that it permits, guides, limits and/or resists specific motions and prevents other specific motions.[2] Of necessity, the exact motion to be denied AND the precise motion to be assisted or resisted must be clear. The range of motion desired must also be defined.

Of necessity, some hinging is incorporated as well as a source of external power. An intrinsic power source involves the patient's muscles, whereas an external power source involves rubber bands, springs, tension bars, and so on. Electronic electrical sources of power for replacement of motor function are being used in a current experimental venture with some success.[2]

Dynamic splints are used to overcome gravity, correct muscle imbalance, prevent or correct contractures, correct deformities, replace lost motor function, or strengthen (as an exerciser of weakened muscle forces).

CONSTRUCTION OF THE SPLINT

Many materials are available for constructing the intended splint. These include plaster, plastics, fiberboard, nylon fabrics, and metal. No precise model can be described as each splint must be molded to the individual, contoured to the precise anatomical site, and constructed to achieve the intended goal.

Some general principles should be used in the construction. The splint should be as simple as possible. It should be light in weight, durable, comfortable, easy to keep clean, and cosmetically acceptible to the patient. The patient should be clearly informed as to its application, and be competent to understand its application and principles. Functions of daily living should be encouraged as much as the medical problem permits.

The attachment of splints requires straps or bands. These should never press upon a nerve or blood vessel nor be so constrictive as to cause edema or nerve pressure.

EXAMPLES OF SPLINT TYPES

Numerous types of splint will be illustrated (Figs. 10–1 to 10–15) but it must be remembered that these can only be viewed as illustrating principles of construction[4] that must accomplish a specific function.[5]

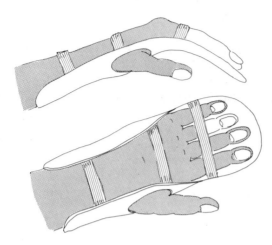

Figure 10–1. Static (rest) splint. This splint can be made of plaster, plastic, Polysar, orthoplast, or other materials and strapped with leather, Velcro, or webbing. It maintains the wrist and fingers in a physiologic position. Among its uses, it is valuable in managing wrist drop from peripheral neuropathies and early flaccid stage of stroke. It prevents deformity, relieves pain, and avoids overstretching of flail musculature.

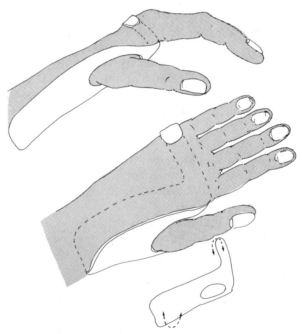

Figure 10–2. Wrist rest splint. This splint can be used as a rest or a semidynamic splint. Its purpose is to maintain the wrist in slight extension, yet permit and assist finger and thumb movement. It can be made of any material. It has definite value in treating median nerve compression (carpal tunnel syndrome).

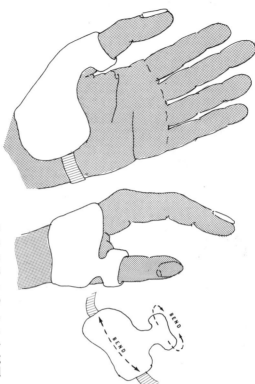

Figure 10-3. Semidynamic thumb splint. This splint is valuable in a flail thumb or in degenerative painful arthritis of the carpometacarpal joint. It immobilizes the thumb in abduction and opposition, permitting tip-to-tip pinch. It has value in spasticity (cerebral palsy), in treating thumb-in-palm, or adducted thumb position.

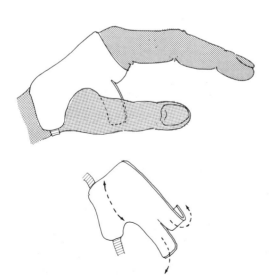

Figure 10-4. Static and semidynamic splint for thumb. This splint mainly maintains thumb in abducted position but does not immobilize the position at the carpometacarpal joint. It may be of value in mild spasticity to decrease thumb-in-palm position.

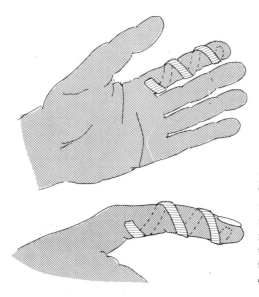

Figure 10-5. Finger rest splint. This simple wrap-around splint uses flexible or plastic material to rest or to maintain gained range of motion in contracture. It provides rest in post-traumatic or degenerative joint changes.

Figure 10-6. Dynamic splint. This type of dynamic splint extends the metacarpophalangeal joint(s). By the power pull of the rubber bands, the proximal phalanx is extended on the metacarpal. There is constant pull while it is being worn. This splint can be used to exercise and strengthen the proximal flexors.

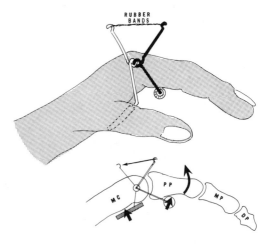

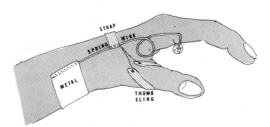

Figure 10-7. Dynamic splint for wrist drop, radial nerve palsy. Using spring wire as a power source, this simple splint extends the wrist and simultaneously abducts the thumb. It is used in radial nerve or nerve root palsies.

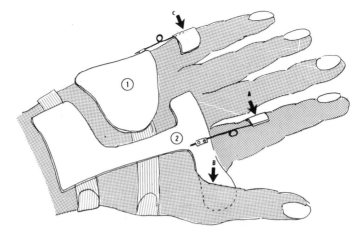

Figure 10–8. Composite dynamic splint, first dorsal interosseous (A), fifth adduction (C). Two spring-wire splints are shown. One (1) adducts the fifth finger and another (2) assists the first dorsal interosseous-index abduction. (B) A flange abducts the thumb. Usually, only one of these splints is worn, or both can be incorporated into one wristband.

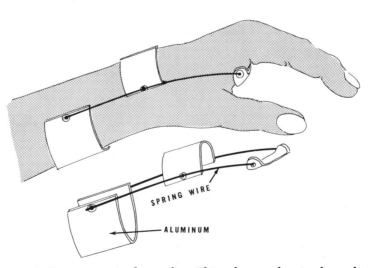

Figure 10–9. Dynamic wrist-drop splint. This splint can be simply made from spring wire and molded aluminum and is an example of the numerous materials that can be employed in making splints.

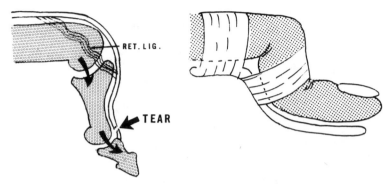

Figure 10–10. Rationale of treatment for mallet finger. Flexing middle phalanx and extending the distal digit permits the extensor tendon to unite. This position pulls the extensor mechanism distally and relaxes the lateral bands.

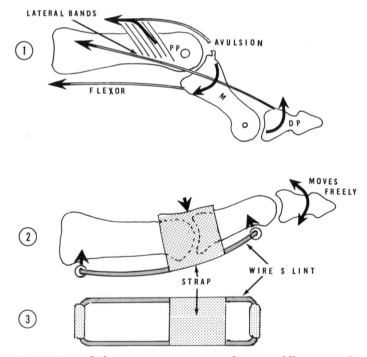

Figure 10–11. Buttonhole rupture, extensor tendon at middle joint, split treatment. (1) Avulsion of the extensor tendon permits the lateral bands to move in a palmar direction, pulling in a proximal direction. The flexor tendons now flex the middle phalanx (MP) and the lateral bands extend the distal phalanx (DP). (2) The splint is made of firm wire bent to extend the middle joint. The strap is inelastic. The distal phalanx is left free and motion is encouraged. (3) Dorsal view of the splint.

Figure 10-12. Isoplast isoprene splint. Models are made in several-size patterns for immediate application. The plastic is heated by hot water or heat gun, then cut and molded easily to the patient's hand. (Adapted from Willis B: The use of orthoplast isoprene splints in the treatment of the acutely burned child. Am J Occup Ther 23:57, 1969.)

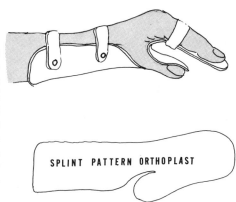

SPLINT PATTERN ORTHOPLAST

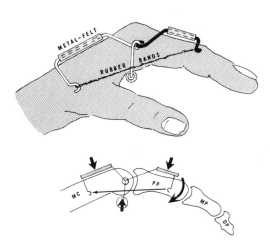

Figure 10-13. Dynamic splint to flex metacarpophalangeal joint, Bunnell knuckle breaker splint. This dynamic splint powered by rubber bands flexes the metacarpophalangeal joint that is contracted following fracture, dislocation, burns, Volkmann's ischemic contracture, and the like. These splints are commercially available.

Figure 10-14. Dynamic splint, post-operative in Dupuytren's contracture. Following palmar fasciotomy in Dupuytren's contracture the digital extension can be maintained by the above splint which permits use of the hand and thumb and first two digits free.

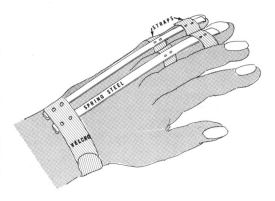

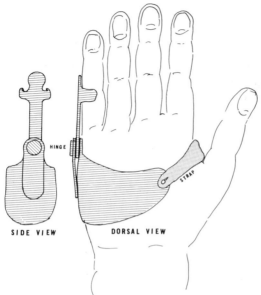

HINGE

STRAP

SIDE VIEW   DORSAL VIEW

Figure 10–15. Dynamic ulnar deviation splint (University of Michigan).

Many have already been described for specific conditions in previous chapters.

As time passes new materials are becoming available and a new techniques of hand rehabilitation are also evolving. The dynamics of hand functions are being studied[6] and researched.[7] The future of hand rehabilitation requires knowledge and experience in all of the above.

REFERENCES

1. Schultz-Johnson K: Splinting–a problem solving approach. In Stanley BG, Tribuzi SM (eds): Concepts in Hand Rehabilitation. FA Davis, Philadelphia, 1992, pp 238–271.
2. Licht S (ed): Orthotics Etcetera (Physical Medicine Library, Vol 9). Elizabeth Licht, New Haven, Conn., 1966.
3. Anderson M: Functional Bracing of the Upper Extremities. Charles C Thomas, Springfield, Ill., 1948.
4. Bunnell S.: Splinting the Hand. American Academy of Orthopedic Surgery Instructional Course Lecture 9:233, 1952.
5. Redford JB, Giewish G, Jiminez J: Simple Splints, Principles and Techniques, University of Alberta Hospital, Edmonton, Alberta, Canada, 1969.
6. Brand PW: Clinical Biomechanics of the Hand. CV Mosby, St. Louis, 1985, pp 106–107.
7. Fess EE, Phillips C: Hand Splinting: Principles and Methods, ed 2. CV Mosby, St. Louis, 1987, pp 137 and 234.

Index

A "t" following a page number indicates a table; an "f" following a page number indicates a figure.

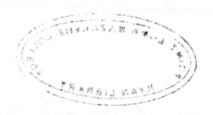